No Fat Chicks

No Fat Chicks

How Big Business
Profits by Making Women
Hate Their Bodies—
and How to Fight Back

Terry Poulton

A Birch Lane Press Book
Published by Carol Publishing Group

A Birch Lane Press Book
Published by Carol Publishing Group
Birch Lane Press is a registered trademark of Carol
Communications, Inc.

Editorial, sales and distribution, and rights and permissions inquiries
should be addressed to Carol Publishing Group, 120 Enterprise
Avenue, Secaucus, N.J. 07094.

In Canada: Canadian Manda Group, One Atlantic Avenue, Suite
105, Toronto, Ontario M6K 3E7

Carol Publishing Group books may be purchased in bulk at special
discounts for sales promotion, fund-raising, or educational purposes.
Special editions can be created to specifications. For details, contact
Special Sales Department, Carol Publishing Group, 120 Enterprise
Avenue, Secaucus, N.J. 07094.

Manufactured in the United States of America
10 9 8 7 6 5 4 3 2 1

Library of Congress Cataloging-in-Publication Data

Poulton, Terry.
    No fat chicks : how big business profits by making women hate their
    bodies—and how to fight back / Terry Poulton.
        p. cm.
    "A Birch Lane Press book."
    Includes bibliographical references and index.
    ISBN 1-55972-423-4
    1. Weight loss. 2. Weight loss preparations industry. 3. Women—
    Health and hygiene. 4. Body image. 5. Overweight women.
    I. Title.
    RM222.2.P67   1997
    613'.04244—dc21   97-19002
                                                                  CIP

For my godchildren, Michael Paauw and Amelia Jackson Purdy, and my littlest nieces and nephew, Elise, Brittany, Emma, and Nathan, with hope that they'll always think for themselves

And in loving memory of Lesley Paauw Cox

Contents

No Fat Chicks

1

Discovering a Billion-Dollar Brainwash

....

One morning, Kate and Cindy and Claudia and all the other fashion models in New York suddenly received pink slips from their modeling agencies. "Sorry, babe. But your brand of lanky, long-legged beauty is obsolete. Ciao!"

Kate and Cindy and Claudia and all the other fashion models in New York galloped to the nearest newsstand—and discovered, to their horror, that it was true! A thousand magazine covers had been launched by a valentine-faced thirteen-year-old who stood just four feet tall and weighed only fifty-five pounds. She was Scottish and came from the latest cultural mecca, Flinging Edinburgh.

Her name was McScrawny.

At first, the American fashion world had been aghast. But recognizing a lucrative bandwagon when it oom-pah-pah-ed along, they hopped aboard and began singing McScrawny's praises morning, noon, and night. And decreeing—for everyone who's anyone, darling—the teensy tartan ensembles that complemented her miniature charms to be the height of fashion.

Soon it became impossible to stroll down a street, open a magazine, snap on a TV set, go to a movie, glance in a store window, or glimpse a billboard without seeing images of McScrawny. She became every-one's ideal.

Meanwhile, Kate and Cindy and Claudia and millions upon millions of other American women sank into a deep depression. Not only did they look terrible in tam-o'-shanters, they just couldn't measure up—or rather down—to McScrawny. Yet their every waking moment was bombarded by messages that any woman larger than McScrawny was unforgivably disgusting, grossly unlovable, and utterly worthless.

So they begged their doctors to chop five or six inches from their shins. They clamored for a waist-cinching operation in which the bottom ribs are removed to produce a true wasp waist. They paid electrolysists fortunes to reshape their hairlines to match McScrawny's deep widow's peak. They bought every pill, potion, gadget, and gizmo they could get their hands on. Some forced themselves to throw up nearly every morsel they ate. Some smoked their heads off. Some popped the diet drugs that suddenly began appearing in stores, plus laxatives, diuretics, and amphetamines as if they were vitamins. And—it goes without saying—they dieted and exercised frantically.

But nothing worked. The harder the woebegone women tried to shrink themselves to McScrawny's size, the more stubbornly their bodies resisted.

Just to make it worse, they couldn't find any decent clothes. They simply weren't being made anymore in sizes larger than 1. Which left nothing but the dowdy duds at down-market shops that made them feel they'd died and gone to Polyester Purgatory.

No employer would hire them. No doctor or lawyer or butcher or baker or corporate chief would treat them respectfully. No one wanted to date them, let alone walk them down the aisle. The husbands and children who were acquired before McScrawnymania were ashamed to be seen with them.

And their images were nowhere to be found in the mass media. In fact, the only time they *were* paid any attention, it was to mock them. After all, what could be more ridiculous than weighing over fifty-five pounds, measuring above four feet, or being beyond your teens?

All the females in the land—except for the .0001 percent who were naturally McScrawnyesque—came to hate themselves, despise each other, and meekly accept the rising tide of contempt being orchestrated against them, day by day, pound by pound, dollar by dollar.

Then one day the madness simply stopped.

Poof!

Kate and Cindy and Claudia and all the other women in the land awoke from the evil trance and said to themselves: "This is stupid. It's wrecking my life.

"Let McScrawny look like McScrawny. And I'll look like myself."

Preposterous? Yes. But only the "poof" part is pure fantasy. Much of this parable has actually occurred since 1967, when American women became obsessed with becoming as ultra-thin as a teenaged fashion model named Twiggy, who'd just arrived from Swinging London. Since then, even women who wouldn't dream of mutilating their shins, ribs, or hairlines succumbed, to one extreme or another, to a new Eleventh Commandment: Thou Shalt Not Be Fat.

For most of my life, I was one of these desperate dieters. In fact, my obsession actually made me famous. How? Like Oprah Winfrey, I promised an entire country that I'd lose weight, and did so in a glaring spotlight, only to regain it. Then, also like Oprah, I learned from personal experience that hell is having to show up fat when *everyone* knows you're supposed to be thin.

She handled it by wailing to her tearstained diary about how disgusted she was with herself. I tried something a little goofier while regaining the sixty-five pounds millions of magazine readers had watched me whittle away during an arduous six-month stint of practically camping out in a gym, living on carrot sticks and little else.

From coast to coast, my "Chronicles of the Incredible Shrinking Terry" attracted affectionate fan letters and resulted in my photos being plastered on fridge doors and gym bulletin boards. After a lifetime as a wallflower, I was a hero to every woman who ever longed to be slim.

And then my pet albatross came flapping back to its longtime roost (just as these tenacious birds do to at least 95 percent of all dieters). I was a freelance magazine writer in the media-savvy city of Toronto, where all my colleagues knew to the pound what I was supposed to weigh. As I rapidly reinflated, I tried toiling as much as possible by phone and memo, but eventually I had to show up for editorial meetings.

That's when I hatched a gambit worthy of Lucy Ricardo at her ditzi-est. Instead of wearing a warm winter coat, I flung a big green cape over my prediet raincoat. Then, whenever I made an entrance, I dra-matically swirled the cape off and remained hidden (I hoped) inside my raincoat. If any of my colleagues caught on, they were kind enough not to squeal.

Today I can finally laugh at my transparent ploy instead of cringing from a sense of failure that's dogged me since childhood. But there was nothing funny about the physical and psychological privations I suffered during my magazine marathon. Or the awful lifelong struggle that preceded it. Or feeling like a fraud even while taking a very pub-lic bow for achieving my goal.

For more than a decade afterward, I had no idea why I felt so guilty and haunted by what others regarded as an inspirational piece of writ-ing. Now I've finally figured it out. It was because I never questioned whether I actually wanted to obliterate a third of my physical self. Not when a leading magazine asked me to do so, and not for the twenty-five years when I dieted so obsessively on my own. Neither did any-one else. It was just a given that women must be thin.

Yet even while wasting so much time, energy, money, and self-esteem trying to obey, subconsciously I was rebelling. A part of me always knew that people must hold tight to their real identity—what-ever it happens to be—and refuse to be squashed to fit any phony, oppressive standard of acceptability. Ignoring this fundamental wisdom by doing my diet series meant betraying myself and everyone I'd influ-enced into blind conformity.

"No one can make you feel inferior without your consent," Eleanor Roosevelt once wrote. Somewhere inside, I knew I'd given my consent to conferring inferior status on not only overweight women, but every-one else who embodies something—anything—our society denigrates.

This realization sank in only after many subsequent spins on the diet carousel, a stomach-stapling operation, and many more years of misery. When I finally understood it, I began achieving what I had really wanted all along: respect, from myself and from others.

What I vowed would be my "diet to end all diets" was set in motion by editors at *Chatelaine*—Canada's top women's magazine—who knew about my Sisyphean, totally typical, lifelong battle with excess weight. Although I was never a compulsive binge eater, I led a habitually sedentary life and ate too many sweet, carbohydrate-laden comfort foods. That, plus decades of yo-yo weight levels, slowed my metabolism and strip-mined my body of fat-burning muscle tissue. Like many of the estimated one-third of American women who are overweight— and the 89 percent who believe they're too heavy—I'd been on dozens of diets and lost and regained hundreds of pounds.

Before then, I'd had a lucky start as a precocious, pretty, and beloved child growing up in western Canada. But I lost my "golden girl" status when I began gaining weight in prepubescence after our single-parent family moved to a strange town and my mother began working outside the home. It seemed as if all the love in my life had suddenly disappeared. The only ways I knew to comfort myself were reading and eating, and I began doing plenty of both. Soon none of my good qualities seemed to count anymore, as praise and friendship were replaced by taunts and ostracism. Photos of me as a teenager don't look all that bad, but I felt like a monster.

By the time I reached my twenties, bag-of-bones Twiggy had replaced curvy Marilyn Monroe as the reigning standard of beauty. I was so desperate to conform to the increasingly narrow parameters of attractiveness that, by my thirties, I had tried even such extreme measures as noxious daily injections (which compelled me to crave raw meat!) and consuming nothing but liquid protein for five months, à la Oprah and with even worse results, as I wound up losing my gallbladder. Every method worked. But, like determined homing pigeons, the pounds I lost always found their way back. And through the years, my weight crept up while my self-respect sank lower and lower.

Enter my editorial chums at *Chatelaine*. They would pick up the tab for sending me to nutritional, fitness, and psychological counseling if I would promise to lose sixty-five pounds and write about my experiences along the way.

It seemed like every woman's dream. After all, who hasn't experienced the "if only" syndrome? We think, "If only I had the money for a personal chef and trainer, plus a free fitness center to go to for the daily workout. Then I could get in shape and my life would be perfect." Seduced by my "if only" dream, I had no idea I was beginning the toughest and loneliest time of my life, in which I would force-march myself through my own private boot camp, trying to meet the scariest deadline of my career.

At first, the pounds came off steadily as I trudged and ached my way along, remaining mostly faithful to my prudent eating and exercising plan. If I just kept on losing a little over ten pounds a month, I'd have it made. But I fell off the wagon one month while traveling, and hit a plateau during another. Shortly after the halfway point, a fear that was bubbling below my consciousness burst into full-blown terror. I still had forty pounds to lose and only three months until the deadline.

I was in big trouble.

What no one really understood back then was how implacably the human body is programmed to fight when it perceives famine conditions like those I had imposed upon myself during and before my magazine diet. The less I ate and the more I pushed my body to expend energy, the more stubbornly it slowed my metabolism. In other words, it wasn't so much pigging out but starving that created and sustained my excess body fat. If I were a cave woman who couldn't find food, this fail-safe system would have kept me alive. Instead, with the whole country watching, I was headed for the worst failure of my life.

Defeat or drastic measures were my only options, and characteristically, I chose the latter. First, I pleaded with my editors to extend my deadline by a month, arguing that this would show readers just how tough it is to lose so much weight so quickly, even with professional help. But, locked into irrevocable publishing schedules, they refused. So, to be closer to the fitness center, which was twenty miles from our home, I walked out on the man I'd been planning to marry, promising to return when I reached my goal. Instead, I ended up losing the love of my life.

Meanwhile, I was alone in a shabby apartment with nothing but a single chair and a mattress on the floor. In the kitchen, I kept only skim milk and coffee. My nutritionist had forbidden caffeine, but without it, I had no energy at all. To beat the crowd, I hit the gym every morning at about six-thirty, and worked out for at least an hour amid disapproving stares from skinnier patrons. Exhausted, red-faced, and breathless, I would then shower, dress, stumble to my car, and race to

Toronto to work on writing projects. I had no extra time for family, friends, or anything but the all-consuming need to meet my deadline.

At the end of days during which I often ate as few as half of my prescribed 1,000–1,200 calories, I would zip back to the gym, repeat my morning's workout, and then swim twenty-two laps in the Olympic-size pool. Sometimes sleep brought blessed oblivion afterward; sometimes I tossed all night, counting not sheep but regrets. The following day, and the day after that, I would do it all again.

Then I'd write another segment of my diet series in the sunny style that, in retrospect, seems like blatant lying. At the time, though, it seemed as if the upbeat, positive tone, which satisfied my editors' instructions, helped hide the tatters in my pride, and conformed with society's agenda, was my only option. "Because my diet and exercising have brought such good results," I trilled in a typical prevarication, "my general attitude and self-image have improved tremendously and I'm almost constantly euphoric."

With just a few weeks left before my deadline, another magazine assigned me a feature story on a woman whose lifelong obsession with becoming thin actually killed her. As I listened to the testimony at her inquest and realized that her struggles were only slightly more extreme than mine, I became frightened about the possible consequences of my regimen. Even worse was a dawning suspicion that in my hell-bent effort to get slim, I was squandering the gift of just being alive. If I hadn't been so publicly committed to my diet, I would have quit. Instead, I persevered.

And then, in June of 1982, there I was, a beaming "cover girl," sixty-five pounds lighter and suddenly a media star. As I drifted from microphone to camera to tape recorder, I tried to ignore an inner sense of turmoil that grew with every tactless, backhanded compliment that revealed the contempt in which I had previously been held. Keep smiling, I remember telling myself. You've won. You're finally giving them what they always demanded. They're finally giving you what you were really starving for: not food, but acceptance.

Yet a voice somewhere inside kept shrieking that there was something ugly about all this admiration. Where were these people before I bought their approval with hunger pangs, sore muscles, and dread? Why couldn't they see I was merely the same worthwhile person I had always been? How dare they force me—and every other woman—in the words of a Leonard Cohen song, "to go begging in beauty's disguise"?

Anger, ambivalence, and disappointment soon drove me back to comfort food, a sedentary life, and the inevitable consequences of regained weight and renewed despair. Even during the next few years, in the glamorous role of a TV columnist at the *Toronto Star*, interviewing celebrities and jetting to Hollywood and New York, I felt as guilty and scorned as ever. Little by little, I withdrew from my family and friends and plummeted from being a famous writer with a million readers a week into existing as a near-hermit. I was on the run, subconsciously trying to escape the feeling that I had made a colossal mistake.

Seven years ago, I left my longtime home in Toronto for Louisville, Kentucky, without really understanding what was compelling me to "run to nowhere," as I put it at the time. Ostensibly, it was to be near my sister and her family, especially my two-year-old godson. But that was actually secondary. The truth was, I felt like an outcast, so I became one. I'd never married or had children of my own. I'd just put my personal life on hold until I could be thin. Why? Because being overweight meant personifying what society considers the worst disgrace of all for women. And the conflict created by feeling "right" about my essential self, but being unanimously condemned as "wrong," paralyzed me emotionally.

Then, from out of nowhere, a literary agent tracked me down and urged me to write a book about being fat in a society that demands thin. At first, I refused. That book has already been written, I said, citing such excellent works as Susie Orbach's pioneering *Fat Is a Feminist Issue* and Kim Chernin's *The Obsession: Reflections on the Tyranny of Slenderness*. But as I thought more about it and did some serious research, I found the key that unlocked the psychological prison in which I'd wasted most of my life.

The key is money.

In fact, what I ultimately discovered is that the whole diet phenomenon is not about beauty or how much women weigh at all. It's about how much we can be persuaded to spend trying to be thin. The entire process is just a despicable scheme to guarantee annual sales of weight-loss products and services currently estimated at $50 billion in the United States alone.

The biggest tip-off to the truth of this theory is that the women who are the most deluded of all are the millions who are not fat—by any stretch of imagination *except* that of the antifat profiteers. Yet these women truly believe they are too heavy and that they have an obligation to lose that weight by whatever means possible.

When I understood the enormity of this deliberate manipulation of perception, emotion, and prejudice, a horrifying word began rocketing around in my mind: "brainwashing." Was the term too strong, or just right, I wondered? I raced to double-check it in several dictionaries. And came up with precise corroboration:

Brainwashing: 1. A method for changing attitudes or beliefs, especially through torture, drugs, or psychological techniques. 2. Any method of controlled indoctrination.

Given the enormity of the mass deception, the name for what I was dealing with was suddenly obvious. It was nothing less than a "billion-dollar brainwash."

Following the Money

Satisfied that I had rightly perceived the nature of the beast I was battling, I began my research with two basic questions: Where did the wholly artificial idea that all women must be thin come from? And how has the obsessive pursuit of this dubious "ideal" affected not just large women like me, but everyone else in our society?

Surely, I assumed, ample objective data must exist about something millions of people pursue obsessively nearly every day of their lives. But time and time again, my search for answers to straightforward questions led me to virtual black holes. Considering that my topic was anything but arcane, it wasn't just maddening to learn how little reportorial, academic, and governmental attention had been paid; it was shocking. And what I did manage to discover—after researching not only traditional avenues and consulting appropriate authorities, but also soliciting first-person material via (among other methods) queries on the Internet and a classified ad in *USA Today*—is vastly different from what we've all been led to believe.

For starters, waiflike thinness is strictly a twentieth-century concept. In fact, actress Lillian Russell, who was considered the most desirable woman of the 1890s, weighed two hundred voluptuous pounds. Paintings of other abundantly endowed beauties still grace gallery walls all over the world, still draw droves of admirers, and still fetch enormous prices. For centuries, in fact, these robust images, with all the flesh and curves that nature designed, have symbolized the essence of "Woman."

Yet in the 1990s, if any of these renowned beauties were somehow to step out of her frame and waft from her time to ours, she would find herself not beloved, but virtually demonized. She would have difficulty obtaining something as ephemeral as a date or as fundamental as a husband. Or a good job. Or equal legal protection. Or first-class health care. Or a good education. Or decent clothing. Or basic human respect.

Today, like the millions of American women who resemble her, she'd be denounced as an offender of a tyrannical new commandment. A legal and social taboo in any other context, it bellows through all the mass media, from haute couture magazines to the crude common denominator of bumper stickers: NO FAT CHICKS!

True, the "ideal" feminine figure has expanded and contracted, been pushed, pulled, wrapped, strapped, and caged throughout history. Society imperiously demands that women contort their bodies to fit the current fashions. Women sheepishly comply, and everyone praises them for doing so.

And over and over again, psyches are manipulated by diverse commercial and cultural factions not only to physically fixate on the new image, but to imbue her with all manner of positive spiritual qualities. Simultaneously, those who least epitomize her are assigned sinister attributes and punished accordingly, with measures ranging from derision to exclusion to economic privation.

C'est la vie? Just one of human nature's inevitable games? Definitely. But in our day, the game has been fixed. As profitable as it has always been to wager on the wayward gusts of fashion, there was a fortune waiting for anyone who could know for certain which way the next wind would blow. And then keep it whistling exactly that way.

But how?

By creating a cash cow, coercing all females into wanting to look just like her, and then selling them the myriad products necessary to recreate her image. That the quest would prove impossible for most women guaranteed everlasting profits.

The bovine imagery seems ludicrous when applied to a gangly, ninety-one-pound English model named Twiggy. Yet since her debut in 1967, when she became the darling of the fashion world and the incongruous ideal of nearly everyone else, her image—and that of latter-day clones like Kate Moss—has been milked for billions. During the first decade after Twiggy's debut, the annual take from the labyrinthine American antifat industry soared to $10 billion, 95 percent of which was spent by women. And in the following decades, that total has *quintupled*.

Thanks to this "billion-dollar brainwash," our culture's ideas about beauty have become more irrational than ever before—so irrational that

- most Americans alive today have no memory of a time when thinness was *not* a national obsession, and thus regard the artificial as normal;
- the average weight of the models, actresses, and beauty pageant contestants we are urged to imitate has plunged to at least 25 percent lower than that of the average American woman;
- nearly 30,000 women stated, in the largest such survey to date, that they'd rather lose weight than achieve *any* other goal—despite the fact that only 25 percent were overweight and another 25 percent were actually underweight;
- millions of women are so terrified of being fat they choose to court disaster by smoking and abusing laxatives, diuretics, and amphetamines to stay thin; and thousands of teenagers eschew birth control pills for the same reason, resulting in a sizable percentage of the millions of babies born to unwed parents;
- formerly fat women say that, rather than regain their weight, they would deliberately choose to be blind, deaf, or have a limb amputated;
- the annual mortality rate attributable to desperate weight-loss practices, including thousands of drastic surgeries, probably numbers in the thousands, yet goes unnoticed;

• no one has realized that eating disorders have reached such epidemic numbers that there are now 50 times more women in North America suffering from anorexia and bulimia than are living with AIDS;
• 11 percent of the respondents in a recent survey said that if genetic predisposition to obesity was identified in their unborn children, they would opt for abortion.

What all this has meant to large women like me, who are the antithesis of Twiggy, is anguishing social marginalization. Our consequent attempts to conform with the narrow new parameters of acceptability have been nothing short of barbaric.

We have had our jaws wired shut, our stomachs stapled, and yards of our intestines hacked off. We've had chunks of ourselves liposuctioned away. We've had our derrieres injected with HCG (a noxious concoction containing the urine of pregnant women). And we've existed for months at a time on a gooey "protein-sparing" powder partly composed of cattle hooves.

We've starved, binged, and vomited. We've jogged and rowed and bench-pressed and stair-stepped ourselves into exhausted stupors. We've ingested appetite suppressants, metabolism accelerators, dangerous diuretics, and innumerable other snake-oil placebos.

Some of us have died. Our death certificates probably specified something such as heart irregularity or exhaustion. But the real cause was suicide, accidental or deliberate, because the victims had so thoroughly internalized society's disgust that their self-loathing proved lethal.

Many of us who survived accepted punishment as if we really were criminals. We condemned ourselves to a prison of shame and threw away the key, psychologically suspending our lives until the elusive day when we would be validated by thinness.

Ironically, just before the Twiggy phenomenon began reshaping millions of bodies and torturing millions of psyches, the reigning feminine ideal was epitomized by a buxom blond movie star. She had billowy hips, a pillowy belly, and more than a hint of womanly thigh. Her name was Marilyn Monroe and she made Twiggy look like a popsicle stick. Yet today Marilyn probably couldn't even get an audition.

And in the subsequent three decades since Twiggy displaced Marilyn, women and girls of all sizes have felt so forced into trying to duplicate the emaciated image that they've hated themselves when they failed the next-to-impossible task.

Brainwashed by inescapable, advertising-driven messages worthy of an Orwellian nightmare, women of all ages, and from all strata of society, feel obliged to disregard the individuality of their physiques and circumstances, and to squander their self-esteem, relationships, money, time, health, and sometimes even their lives.

No one really asks why.

No one asks how today's women, whose eyes were opened to modern female subjugation by the 1963 publication of Betty Friedan's *The Feminine Mystique*, could possibly have knuckled under to a dictum that's as oppressive as ancient Chinese foot-binding.

No one asks why doctors—physical and psychological—who should know the overwhelming odds against the average woman ever sustaining Twiggy's bag-of-bones look, buy into the delusion, are bought off by profiteers, or hop aboard the money wagon themselves.

No one asks why public health officials turn a blind eye to the lucrative lunacy. Or why otherwise enlightened organizations and employers, after finally recognizing alcoholism and insanity as diseases rather than sins or character flaws, callously blame and mistreat the overweight.

Even when belated attention is paid to the eating disorders and emotional problems of thin women, fat women remain beyond the pale. No one called a halt, even when potentially eye-opening data began drifting in about the body's set-point mechanism, the adverse metabolic effect of food deprivation, the unalterable modus operandi of fat cells, the lethal risks of yo-yo weight levels, genetic destiny, and the 95–98 percent failure rate of dieting.

Instead, loving parents blithely allow the No Fat Chicks propaganda to simultaneously warp the sexual and romantic appetites of their sons and to savage the psyches of their daughters, who now fret about their weight in kindergarten and diet from age seven on.

And compassionate people, who abhor every other kind of bigotry, fail to scream bloody murder against the epidemic of prejudice attacking all females who look more like Lillian and Marilyn than Twiggy and Kate.

Result? While our loved ones urge us onward, women and girls stampede to enrich the profiteers, who gleefully build their "billion-dollar brainwash" on the reprehensible bedrock of instilled shame and choreographed contempt.

When I finally saw how this gigantic scam works, the shame I had felt for a lifetime turned into boiling outrage at the way bogus "beauty" imperatives impoverish individual women's lives and confound our collective progress toward equality. Simultaneously, I learned about the evolution of metabolic programming and realized it isn't always overeating that keeps people fat. More often, it is punitive, prolonged dieting that trains our bodies to hold on to every pound. This double epiphany literally liberated me from a lifetime of obsession and shame.

It also ignited an ambition to inspire the biggest jail break in history. I now know that no one has to wait until losing X number of pounds before escaping the prison of psychological pain and coercive constriction. We can all bust out immediately, simply by understanding how the profiteers brainwash women to hate their bodies—and everyone to forget that nature creates people in a rich variety of shapes and sizes. Only when they're free of the supremely stupid and corrupt No Fat Chicks delusion can "overweight" women stop accepting inferior status and start feeling empowered to do what's best for their bodies and their lives.

Am I promoting unhealthy obesity in this book? On the contrary. I know very well that too many of us weigh too much, and exercise too little, for our own good. Nothing in *No Fat Chicks* is meant to deny that reality. But the fact is, the current epidemic of obesity cannot simply be chalked up to "couch potato-ism." Other leading causes of excess weight are our culture's evolution toward sedentary work and leisure lifestyles, and the high fat and sugar content in modern convenience foods (which, it should be remembered, also liberated women from long, laborious hours in the kitchen).

The *major* culprits in many, many cases—including my own—are the antifat profiteers themselves. What makes them culpable? The fact that they've duped us into the incessant dieting that actually creates and sustains obesity by wrecking the metabolism, robbing the body of fat-burning muscle tissue, and inducing a physical and psychological need to binge. What better way could there possibly be to guarantee profits in perpetuity than to persuade us to keep on keeping on with never-ending diets?

This book is primarily about mending broken hearts and troubled minds, not about transforming bodies into marvels of fitness. In fact, my ever wise mother suggested making it absolutely clear that it doesn't contain a single diet. She's right. The only reducing advice I want to share is not for your body—because that's entirely your business—but for the heaviness that was deliberately implanted in your heart and soul so that your pocket could be picked.

However, far from being oblivious to physical health, I have found—to my delight and amazement after a lifetime of fighting my weight every step of the way—that when my mental attitude was finally healed, my body automatically began sorting itself out. I have dieted for the last time. And stopped heeding the voices, inside and outside my head, that tell me to despise myself. Yet my attitude toward what I eat and how I treat my body has been transformed, quite effortlessly, into what it should have been during and after my magazine weight-loss series. With coercion out of the picture, I now freely choose whether and how I will work out (it varies depending on my work schedule) and what I eat (mostly vegetables, fruits, and complex carbohydrates with very little fat, plus occasional sweets about which I no longer agonize).

And the happy result is that since my one-woman jail break, I've been losing weight without dieting. The total as of this writing is probably about 50 pounds. But that's just a guess because I've promised myself never to step on a scale again, let alone allow it to measure my self-worth.

I don't look like Kate Moss or Twiggy, and I never will. Logically enough, I look a lot more like my grandmother and her stocky German ancestors. But with a reasonable amount of steady effort—which I now *want* to make, for my health and my appearance—I am working on achieving the best possible version of *my own* natural physique.

So when I gaze at my reflection today, whether in a mirror or in other people's eyes, I no longer see the grotesque fun-house distortion that tormented me for so long. Instead, I see what I always wanted to be: not a raving beauty, just a contented, self-respecting, normal person. I'm not slender, but neither is the average American woman, especially in middle age. Nor am I "proud to be fat," as some advocates for the admirable size-acceptance movement declare.

I am just me. And it's finally enough.

But let's say you can't quite accept the scenario I've sketched. Or you think that *some* of it may have happened to *some* women, but only the truly obese. Or maybe you just don't buy a theory as far-fetched as mine, namely, that antifat conspirators make their fortunes by secretly waging campaigns of terror and disinformation worthy of the Kremlin in its heyday. Or that a cabal of strategists straight out of George Orwell's *1984* have made alchemy a reality by creating insecurity and transforming it into gold.

Or perhaps, like so many other people these days, you despise the whole notion of entrapment. We just don't like victims right now, do we? Solution: Make like Marie Antoinette and deny their existence. Or loftily insist that they walked into whatever trap ensnares them with their eyes wide open, so where do they get off complaining about the consequences?

As Dana Carvey's famous Church Lady would say: How conveeeeenient! What better strategy could any would-be billionaire have than to shut the eyes, and quiet the conscience, of an entire nation? The ideology that everyone is personally responsible for their own condition, and that "victims" are just too lazy to pull themselves up by their own bootstraps, or too weak to take the rap for their own failures, is certainly working to keep us from having to spend our money on "losers" like the poor, the elderly, the disabled, downsized workers, single mothers, women who are pregnant against their will, crime victims, homosexuals, or shortchanged minorities. Think it's accidental? Take a look at the rapidly widening income gap between the haves and have-nots in this country, and then think again.

But no matter how little you may agree with my argument, you must be convinced by now that the forces I collectively call the antifat profiteers are smart. They couldn't make $50 billion a year selling things that don't work without being flat-out brilliant.

Wouldn't they also be bright enough to know it's just plain stupid to limit their market to the one-third of American women who truly are overweight? Could any bean counter worth his or her stock options possibly miss the breathtaking potential in snagging, not just fat women, but everyone else? How to do it? By inventing phantom flab where none exists, and then convincing the entire female population that their lives depend on getting rid of it—that they must, and can, attain and sustain the same weight level that nature has conferred on just 5 percent of them, if they just buy the right products.

So maybe we *can* agree that, in a spectacular example of capitalism triumphant, senseless traps have been deliberately set. But just a minute here; today's women insist on being treated as intelligent adults. So why should anyone care if they willingly step into such snares? What *about* personal responsibility? Isn't *that* the ultimate answer to nearly every ill we're prey to?

Now that's the right question—the one that's ringing throughout this country just now. And the answer is yes. Personal responsibility *is* the fundamental solution. There's just one problem. If you're drowning, you won't survive long enough to rely on yourself if you can't get your hands on a life preserver. If you're caught in a trap, chewing off your own leg is not the best way to get out.

So the real answer is: First you get free, and *then* you steer your own course, taking care to avoid raging rivers and sharp-toothed traps. In the No Fat Chicks context, as I see it, the life preserver is composed of facts, and that's what I've ferreted out and compiled in this book. *This* is the light I finally saw after a lifetime of delusion. It was powerful enough to wise me up, and I'm certain it can do so for others as well.

But what if you're among the fortunate minority who are naturally slim and unconflicted? Maybe you assume this book is not for you. It is. Why? Because every *other* American woman has been taught to live in fear of the cruelty and discrimination I describe. And even if *you* have managed to resist body image problems and contempt for obesity, how about our daughters, who don't have the psychological fortitude to fight off antifat propaganda? And how about the 11 million young women who are—let's be bold enough to use the "v" word here—victims of eating disorders, and therefore in mortal danger?

And, ultimately, what about our collective future, not just in this country, but on this planet? Isn't it a tantalizing probability that, if millions of women stop being so preoccupied with unattainable "beauty" standards, their time, energy, creativity, and money will be freed up and applied to solving the real problems that confront us? I believe the answer is a resounding yes.

The Beginning of the End

No Fat Chicks necessarily begins by tracing a dark, depressing, and infuriating story. But even a game as astronomically profitable as the billion-dollar brainwash can't last forever. In fact, "time" is already starting to be called by the most powerful team on the field—those wizards of fundamental change, the baby boomers—in ways I never believed I'd live to see.

Just as they rewrote other cultural rules they considered unjust, many are now realizing that the odious schemes of the antifat profiteers must be exposed and resisted. Demographically, most of the boomers are thickening as fast as they're aging. And their priorities have shifted away from frivolous youthful pursuits, such as unrealistic thinness, and toward maturity, practicality, and true physical and psychological health. Many are also outraged by the epidemic of eating disorders afflicting their daughters.

Logical result: The almightiest dollars of all are beginning to reverse the artificially induced, three-decade pandemic of delusion. So the words of the prophets/profits written on the subway walls (to borrow from Simon and Garfunkel) are changing from Thou Shalt Squash Thyself to Thou Shalt Get Real. And the most prescient lifestyle profiteers, from manufacturers to advertisers, have begun trumpeting the desirability of everything from loose-fitting jeans to palatable low- and no-fat food products.

At last, medical reports about the realities of the body's weight imperatives are being heeded. Finally, antidiscrimination organizations such as the National Organization for Women, the American Civil Liberties Union, and the Equal Employment Opportunity Commission are recognizing the inequities affecting society's last scapegoat.

Artists and cultural commentators are starting to explore a theme that's rife with dramatic possibilities. Crusade-loving politicians are recognizing, if not their public responsibility, at least the opportunity to mount a fresh white horse.

And the activism of size acceptance organizations such as the National Association to Advance Fat Acceptance (NAAFA) is finally beginning to attract a glimmer of respectful media attention. The volume of their collective voice is still that of a gnat trying to outshout a baboon, but it shouldn't be long before their influence prevails.

Best of all, some of the primary antifat profiteers are being forced into some serious reducing of their own. Some are even being prodded in a saner direction by federal trade regulators and public health officials. True to form, the chief response of these money-hungry predators was to launch "Operation Waif" (actually, "Twiggy II") to try to get their skinny ducks back in a row. And, when that didn't work, they simply switched gears and deluged women with identical editorial and advertising messages equating fitness with power. But it's obvious that all they're *really* peddling is just more profit-producing insecurity.

I wrote this book to keep them from getting away with it any longer. And to signal the beginning of the end of the detestable No Fat Chicks era; help consign the period to the oblivion it deserves as just another blip on history's time line; provide a step-by-step exposé of how the de facto conspiracy to get rich by stigmatizing large women—and traumatizing the rest of the female population—came about; and to name names and point an accusing finger directly at those who sell shame by the pound and prejudice by the dollar.

My ambitions for No Fat Chicks are threefold. First, I want to inform, dignify, encourage, and empower large women like me by placing the blame where it belongs—not on the victims, but on those who deliberately victimize us and, in the process, coarsen our society to the point of legitimizing cruelty. Doing so will, I am certain, arm the truly overweight with the factual and psychological means to end the merciless barrage of prejudice, exploitation, and discrimination that dogs their days and poisons their lives.

Secondly, I want to help smaller women see the billion-dollar brainwash for the trap it is, and to assist them in liberating themselves—and future generations of children—from its coercive power.

And thirdly, I hope to help men, educators, the medical community, and public health personnel to understand what's really going on and why it's happening.

To be crystal clear about my message, however, I am *not* recommending that anyone ever stop caring about weight control or genuine fitness. This is simply a human necessity, just like taking care of every other aspect of our health. What I *am* saying is that there are better ways of accomplishing this than engaging in expensive, counterproductive, soul-destroying exercises in futility.

Bottom line? I believe that our so-called obsession with thinness is not an implacable cultural phenomenon at all. It's not about being slender, beautiful women. It's about being obedient little consumers. I challenge anyone to come up with a theory that's more plausible than this. And "just sort of happened" doesn't count.

As I march gratefully along the trail blazed by such cultural heroes as Betty Friedan (*The Feminine Mystique*), Naomi Wolf (*The Beauty Myth*), Susan Faludi (*Backlash: The Undeclared War Against American Women*), and Susie Orbach (*Fat Is a Feminist Issue*), I am hoping that *No Fat Chicks* will serve as one more of the scattered pieces of a giant jigsaw puzzle that's gradually revealing the truth about women's lives.

2

The Incredible Shrinking Woman

···

We *think* we think for ourselves. Our eyes are wide open, and we make all our own choices, right? Sorry. If this were true, we wouldn't believe the most preposterous fairy tale ever concocted: that to be fat is to be like Cinderella's stepsisters: ugly, lazy, mean, and stupid; and to be thin is to live happily ever after.

And the kicker is the notion that what bamboozled us into this mass delusion just sort of happened, or that women created it themselves, probably out of our insecurity about storming male bastions. Sure. And I suppose the Davy Crockett coonskin-cap craze of the 1950s also "just happened" and had nothing to do with the marketing genius of Walt Disney!

Here's what really occurred. It's the history we must learn from if we're ever to stop repeating it.

New York, March 20, 1967: The shy, near-skeletal English teenager who jets in on TWA flight 703 looks nothing like the cash cow she is destined to become. Nor do her elfin face and urchin figure (ninety-one pounds on a five-foot, seven-inch frame) identify her as a Trojan horse whose secret mission is to entrap the female population of America for the next three decades.

Reporters loitering at an airport newsstand wait impatiently for the press conference to welcome Lesley Hornby, the seventeen-year-old fashion model who swept to the top of the heap in Swinging London the previous year, despite being so emaciated she was nicknamed Sticks, OxFam, and, ultimately, Twiggy.

Flipping through magazines to pass the time, the journalists find nothing surprising in the photo spreads of popular beauties. Grownups are still in style, and even those who sport the flamboyant new "mod gear" don't look much different from many of the women who amble through the airport. More photogenic, perhaps, but roughly the same age and size as the kind of real-life ladies who've been considered attractive for as long as anyone can remember.

As a bright orange coat and two coltish, miniskirted legs move into view, the world wobbles imperceptibly and starts spinning in a sinister new direction.

In a wacky, six-week whirlwind after Twiggy's arrival at Kennedy Airport, the diminutive cockney "bird" metamorphosed into a mammoth, completely unprecedented marketing phenomenon. Her image was plastered everywhere. Her photo sessions caused near-riots all over Manhattan. Hairstylists duplicated her cropped locks as fast as their scissors could snip. Modeling agencies trampled one another to sign her up. Mannequins matching her 31-22-32 silhouette suddenly appeared in Fifth Avenue windows, hastily clad in the Twiggy Enterprises line of clothing, which was being imported from London at the rate of $500,000 per week.

Before she winged back across the Atlantic, Twiggy was the object of a genuine media frenzy from which not even the stodgy *New York Times* could remain aloof, even though it described her as "just like your next-door neighbor, if he happens to be a skinny twelve-year-old boy." Scribes from *Life, Look, Mademoiselle*, the *Saturday Evening Post*, the *New Yorker, McCall's*, and *Ladies' Home Journal* followed her everywhere. A huge press contingent turned out just to watch her get her famous hair trimmed. *Women's Wear Daily*, even while denouncing Twiggy in a front-page editorial as just "a massive publicity stunt," nevertheless splurged with a sixteen-page feature on her.

The rest of the fashion press positively swooned. At the head of the pack was quirky Diana Vreeland, *Vogue* editor and longtime *doyenne* of haute couture, who gushed that Twiggy was "charming . . . disarming [and] delicious," and booked her for four cover shoots with crème de la crème photographer Richard Avedon. Privately, though, Vreeland opined in a memo that "Twiggy is dreadfully swaybacked . . . [and should be told] to pull in her behind [so we'll] have a glorious girl and not an ill-fed adolescent."

Why the commotion? Timing. There were then more than 30 million teenage girls in America, all eager to spend their allowances on anything that differentiated them from their mothers. With rock and roll fomenting rebellion, baby boomers of both sexes were overthrowing parental dominion. And even though the famous "pig in a python" metaphor had yet to be coined to symbolize the sociological clout of these youngsters, what was obvious was that their spending power amounted to a gold rush for marketers.

Even so, few pundits recognized the revolutionary redefinition of beauty Twiggy represented, nor that, in terms of marketing, she was treading where no mere model had ever gone before. One exception was *Newsweek*, which splashed her on its cover and dubbed her "the first child star in the history of high fashion." While other reporters cracked jokes, *Newsweek*'s anonymous feature writer cut right to the big question: "Whether the Twiggy look will now sweep across the U.S., emaciating American teen-agers as it goes. . . ."

It was the right query, but it underestimated the geography. Girls all over the world began shortening their skirts, lengthening their eyelashes, and cutting back on calories—although not to any alarming degree, because youth was still on their side. But Twiggy's older fashion colleagues hit the panic button. "It was a nightmare, trying to keep up," model Gillian Bobroff recalls in Michael Gross's *Model: The Ugly Business of Beautiful Women.* "I . . . started killing myself . . . I never ate." Statuesque Wilhelmina, a top international model of the day, put herself on what she called the "hummingbird diet," eating only twice a week, with cigarettes and black coffee sustaining her between Sundays, when she had a small steak, and Wednesdays, when she ate "a little bowl of soup . . . or a little piece of cheese on a cracker . . . so I wouldn't get too sick . . ."

Other fashion models, indeed all women whose beauty was their professional stock-in-trade, soon felt pressured into adopting similarly stringent regimens, often augmented by diet pills and bulimic behavior. Two of the most prominent were actresses Jane Fonda—who has admitted suffering a twenty-year eating disorder while trying "to get closer to the bone"—and Sally Field, who developed bulimia in response to feeling "immensely unattractive [because] everybody . . . was Twiggy, except me."

But what's most significant here is that, even in ordinary walks of life, it was only a matter of time before the girls who had found it fairly easy to look like Twiggy—and like the Barbie dolls they'd been collecting since 1959—grew up to be women whose bodies had other plans, but whose minds, by then, had been infiltrated by the message of antifat profiteers: that all women have an obligation to be slim.

If you like historical "if only's," here's a lulu: One year after Twiggy's sensational U.S. debut, something happened in Atlantic City that might have averted, or at least mitigated, the pandemic of physical and spiritual starvation she launched—if the media that covered it hadn't gotten away with one of the most blatant whoppers ever told.

We all know that the bizarre practice of bra burning began at the 1968 Miss America pageant, right? Wrong. The real scoop is that a plucky troupe of pioneering feminists, seeking a way to spotlight their aspirations, staged a demonstration to protest the beauty contest. To explicitly signal their rejection of the phony, constricting trappings of "the feminine mystique," they tossed makeup, hair curlers, steno pads, copies of *Playboy*, high heels, girdles, and bras into what they dubbed a "freedom trash can." They also crowned a sheep as the new Miss America. The demonstration was certainly radical for its time, but the symbolism—and the press releases and media interviews—weren't exactly indecipherable.

Yet how was the protest reported? In a way that not only diminished that specific event, but almost fatally trivialized the women's movement itself. What was set afire that day? Nothing. But that didn't stop reporters from calling the event a "bra burning,"* and saddling feminists with an enduring legacy of ridicule and misunderstanding.

---

*A sloppy parallel to males burning their draft cards to protest the Vietnam War.

If only the demonstrators' wake-up call had reached and influenced massive numbers of women in 1968, *and* been followed by responsible coverage of the issues and inequities at the core of the women's liberation movement, our phenomenal subsequent progress might have included the one crucial victory that still eludes us: namely, the enhancement of women's self-respect enough that we understand how bogus, self-defeating, and socially regressive the "beauty" imperative really is.

Instead, for nearly a decade, all the majority of Americans ever saw or heard were sarcastic, irresponsibly distorted portrayals of "libbers" as hairy-legged, combat-booted, man-hating crazies whose goals couldn't possibly have anything to do with the real lives of women and families.

But the dishonest coverage of the Miss America protest was scarcely the first time women have been lied to or about, with devastating results. Let's backtrack to a time when—unbelievable as it seems in our looks-above-all era—there was no such thing as a tyrannical ideal which all women were pressured to imitate.

From Abundant Reality to "Ideal" Fantasy

Standardized clothing sizes didn't even exist until about 130 years ago. Before then, garments were fitted to individual bodies, not the other way around. Fashion had none of the dictatorial power it has today; it was merely a whimsical indulgence of the well-to-do, who were consequently the only folks with strong ideas about how people "should" look.

For most of recorded history, the only way of documenting the faddish evolution of desirable female forms was through statues and paintings. The oldest known example is a tiny clay figure called the *Woman from Willendorf*, which dates back some thirty thousand years. By modern standards, this Earth Mother is a portly conglomeration of rounded masses adding up to perhaps 250 pounds. The increasingly sophisticated statues that turned up later gave us the "classic" notion of feminine beauty that more or less persists today. But would it surprise you to learn that the measurements of the revered Venus de Milo were 43-31-40?

After Venus's ample "buns of marble," there were many more changes to come before anyone dreamed up today's preposterous "buns of steel." Rosy, rounded buttocks were all the rage in one era, and sloping shoulders in another, while breasts were raised, lowered, and sometimes flattened to accentuate enormous bellies or hips. Meanwhile, waists wandered in and out, desirable body weights bobbed up and down, and many other permutations came and went. The front-runners in this historical parade were the "Rubenesque" damsels whose abundance promised fertility.

But here's the point: The shifts in female body shapes were not real, but merely artists' interpretations. And since mass communication was nonexistent, and art and fashion were almost exclusively the property of the rich, so few people saw these images that their power to dictate arbitrary standards of beauty was negligible.

Then came the Industrial Revolution. Mass manufacturing required a mass market, and when the process was eventually extended to encompass clothing, a new chapter in the story of women's bodies began to be written. By the mid-nineteenth century, technological breakthroughs were revving up the production of textiles and some finished garments for both sexes. But it wasn't until the invention of dressmakers' patterns, by Ellen Butterick in 1863, that the need for standard sizes arose. Even then, it was easy enough for a skilled seamstress to yo-yo her seams in or out, according to the client's proportions, which she did (presumably in diplomatic silence) if she wished to be rehired.

At about the same time, an Englishman named Charles Frederick Worth sailed for Paris, where he came up with a prototype for the salons that gradually nudged dressmaking out of cottages and into shops. This commercialization of the process eroded the concept of catering to just one customer's figure at a time. A marketing as well as a design genius, Worth was ahead of his time in many ways, and with another innovation—employing live mannequins to enticingly parade his gowns through the salon—he bequeathed to the general public the concept of the "ideal" figure.

Tastes changed radically thereafter, with colossal crinolines giving way to bodacious bustles, only to be succeeded by the S-shaped curves of the Gibson Girl. But, as in earlier times, these shifts in the way women seemed to be built were accomplished, not by demanding the actual transmutation of bodies, but by altering the designs of clothing as well as the undergarments that coaxed flesh into whatever shape was currently in style. As cruelly uncomfortable as these corsets and other gadgets undoubtedly were, what was on the way was worse.

Yet live mannequins didn't capture the public's attention very quickly (as hard as this is to believe in the age of the "supermodel"). In fact, looking as much as possible like a marketer's arbitrary ideal wasn't really a consideration for quite some time. It was when the apparel industry began to be dominated by presized, ready-to-wear clothing shortly before the turn of the century that the die was permanently cast. From then on, the wearer would be required to fit the garment instead of vice versa.

The Rise of Women's Magazines

Another decisive event in this abbreviated time line was the advent of a means of communication by which women could be taught what was expected of them, beauty-wise (and later on, in oh so many other ways). This virtual operator's manual was the same thing it is today—the women's magazine.

The first two of these secular bibles were piloted by Sarah Josepha Hale. The year was 1828, the venue was Boston, and the publications were, first, *Ladies Magazine* and, then, *Godey's Lady's Book*. Savvy Sarah told readers early on, in an obvious bid to forestall charges of uppityness, that "husbands may rest assured that nothing found in these pages shall cause [their wives] to . . . encroach upon prerogatives of men."

What did get encroached upon in short order were the dimensions of feminine desirability. Thanks to the sheer novelty of *Godey's Lady's Book*, thin was in for the first time. While Europeans looked on in amazement, "the American craze," which lasted only from about 1830 to 1850, prompted such rampant dieting that reformer Harriet Beecher Stowe complained: "Our willowy girls are afraid of nothing so much as growing stout . . . [and] when we see a woman made as a woman ought to be, she strikes us as a monster."

Sound familiar? There was even a foreshadowing of our current epidemic of eating disorders in an article written by J. A. Brillat-Savarin in the year *Godey's Lady's Book* was founded. He told of a young friend named Louise who, after being teased about her size, put herself on a diet consisting of one glass of vinegar per day. Two months later, she was dead.

All in all, the raison d'être of the earliest women's magazines was identical with that of today's. As *Ms.* founding editor Gloria Steinem reported in a riveting exposé titled *Sex, Lies, & Advertising*, the publications existed, then as now, "to create a desire for products, instruct in the use of products, and make products a crucial part of gaining social approval. . ."

The first of these products was, of course, ladies' clothing, which could now be viewed simultaneously by thousands of far-flung readers. What had been missing for centuries—a way to deliver visual images to masses of potential consumers—had finally arrived. Yet, with photographic reproduction still a few decades in the future, the latest fashions had to be sketched by artists, and their renderings of female figures were too idealized and exaggerated to be taken seriously as edicts on how readers should really look.

The coming of the camera would change all that. Now, as historian Anne Hollander writes in *Seeing Through Clothes*, "Perfect feminine beauty no longer formed a still image, ideally wrought by a Leonardo da Vinci. . . . It had become transmuted into a photograph, a single instant that represented a sequence of instants. . . . For this kind of mobile beauty, thinness was a necessary condition." With the mistaken conviction that cameras cannot lie, it was clear sailing for what came to be called "the tyranny of fashion." From now on, women would feel obliged to remodel their body shape in favor of the prevailing silhouette.

Magazines and Marketers Tie the Knot

Poised on the threshold was another kind of tyranny that would be inimical to women's ability to feel at peace with their bodies: advertising. Even without running ads, the earliest women's magazines had effectively touted wares that complemented their genteel messages about the proper way to conduct one's life. But it wasn't long before nascent marketers spied the potential of women's magazines and came a-courting. When the union between product and vehicle was consummated, as Steinem put it, "for the first time, readers could purchase what a magazine had encouraged them to want."

Periodicals were soon peppered with advertisements, many of which focused on fanciful bodily ills—which snake-oil producers were only too eager to cure. Given the immense popularity of such generously endowed women as Lillian Russell, and the long-standing association of fatness with both physical and financial prosperity, it was no wonder that the "heartbreak of corpulence" would not become an editorial and advertising staple until after the First World War.

Instead, publications were apt to target the opposite condition. Chubbiness was considered so desirable that even the beloved actress Sarah Bernhardt was frequently mocked for being too skinny, and caricatured with her head atop such narrow, cylindrical objects as broomsticks, canes, and snakes. Meanwhile, antislenderness ads, such as one placed in *Woman's Home Companion* in 1908 by a company called Nature's Rival, became common. "Does your form lack normal development?" queried the ad. No problem: "You can display a perfect figure, showing the natural, well-rounded bust form of a beautifully developed woman by using . . . an air form corset waist inflated to any desired size."

But both fashion and advertising did an abrupt about-face as the Roaring Twenties approached, and a number of postwar factors led to the debut of a newfangled, hair-bobbed, beanpole-shaped woman called a flapper. Seemingly overnight, the elaborate coiffures and lush but trussed-up physiques of the Victorian and Edwardian eras came to symbolize a past that had enslaved women for too long. "The hoopskirt, the small waist . . . the artificial helplessness, the wretched discomfort . . . [were] emblazoned in sartorial terms," fumed an equal rights tract dated 1920.

Now looking as "narrow as an arrow," to quote some memorable ad copy, was what it took to signal both attractiveness and women's newly won autonomy. Off went long, cumbersome hair. Up went draggy skirts. Out went Mama's mores. Yet, while the "jazz babies" congratulated themselves for escaping corsets and stays, they overlooked a fundamental contradiction: Achieving the androgynous new contours by binding themselves fore and (if necessary) aft, as well as eating far less than in the past, wasn't exactly a radical improvement.

Why didn't flappers realize this? Chiefly because of the heady feeling of victory that came with winning the right to vote in national elections for the first time in history. But also, to a great extent, because marketers, using the popular-culture vehicles of the day, co-opted and trivialized the women's own emancipation rhetoric, just as their heirs would do during the second feminist wave of the 1970s. Case in point: Women's rights marchers were persuaded to hold up Lucky Strike cigarettes as symbolic "torches of freedom" by Edward Bernays, the generally acknowledged father of public relations, on behalf of the American Tobacco Company. Even the term "flapper"—connoting the pointless flapping-about of a beheaded chicken—was dismissive, as "libber" would be later on.

It may sound overly simplistic to say women were hoodwinked into believing that societal permission to reveal their legs, doff their old-fashioned underwear, and adopt boyish silhouettes equaled all the freedom they needed. But the red herring of superficial cultural concessions worked well enough in both eras to stall political momentum. Consequently, as Anne Hollander noted, "the rapidity with which the new, linear form replaced the more curvaceous one [was] startling." In fact, the flapper craze spread faster than any trend had before, or would again until Twiggy came along.

The accelerant was the newest means of mass influence: the movies, especially those featuring whippet-thin stars like Clara Bow and Mary Pickford. As Jeanine Basinger, author of *A Woman's View: How Hollywood Spoke to Women, 1930–1960*, describes this effect: "Women measure themselves by the cultural norms that are presented to them. What is a woman? How is she supposed to look and act? Movies . . . provided models to answer these questions, and women . . . gobbled them up."

Even more influentially, women's magazines began preaching a stern and—except for the Depression and the war years—unrelenting No Fat Chicks sermon that continues to this day. *Vogue*, for example, scolded in 1918 that "there is one crime against the modern ethics of beauty which is unpardonable; far better it is to commit any number of petty crimes than to be guilty of growing fat."

That same year, *Diet and Health With a Key to the Calories* became the first American best-seller in the weight-loss arena. In it, Los Angeles physician Lulu Hunt Peters advised women who were noticeably wider than arrows that they were "viewed with distrust, suspicion, and even aversion."

What was a woman to do if she was guilty of the new "crime" of corpulence? Why, just flip the pages of her favorite magazine until she found an article or an ad promoting the very latest in reducing schemes, potions, gimmicks, gadgets, and gizmos. Her only problem would be choosing between "quasi-scientific diet programs [including] lemon juice, milk and bananas, special breads and seaweed; patent medicines or 'fat reducers' advertised as Citrophan, Figureoids, Berledets, Allan's Antifat, Rengo, Kellogg's Obesity Food, and Marmola [plus] treatments with special baths, pastes, and thinning salts," according to Joan Jacobs Brumberg's *Fasting Girls: The Emergence of Anorexia Nervosa as a Modern Disease.*

If none of that worked, women took other forms of drastic action, and in such large numbers that, by 1926, medical and public-health authorities had become alarmed enough to convene an Adult Weight Conference. One of the speakers reported a practice that is only too well known seventy years later: "Many of our flappers have mastered the art of eating their cake and yet not having it, inducing regurgitation, after a plentiful meal, either by drugs or mechanical means." And if bulimia didn't do the trick, there was one more dangerous option, also still practiced in the 1990s: smoking. "To keep a slender figure . . . Reach for a Lucky instead of a sweet," advised a raft of 1920s ads for Lucky Strikes cigarettes.*

Whichever weight loss scheme she tried, the modern miss could check her progress by hopping onto one of the new home scales (a million of which were sold by the Detecto company in 1925 alone). And if her new regimen should create an unhealthy pallor, well, it was no longer considered scandalous to wear make up, and buckets of it were now pouring onto the market. In fact, everything a modern woman could possibly want was ostensibly hers for the buying. "We grew up founding our dreams on the infinite promise of American advertising," mused Zelda Fitzgerald, who epitomized the "smart young things" of the Jazz Age. "I still believe that one can learn to play the piano by mail and that mud will give you a perfect complexion."

---

*Lucky Strikes' targeting of women helped the American Tobacco Company leap from third position in 1925 (13.7 billion cigarettes sold) to top brand by 1930 (40 billion sold).

Flappers like Zelda were heartily encouraged to assume that they
had come a long way. But, in terms of inescapable beauty imperatives,
they were actually as reined in by the marketers as were their predecessors, and as their descendants would be three-quarters of a century
later. Meanwhile, the true emancipation sought by the original suf-
fragists remained out of reach.

With supreme irony suggesting that misogynist gods were playing a
cosmic trick on women, both national female suffrage and the trend-
setting Miss America beauty pageant turned up in the same year—
1920. But it wasn't a celestial prank; it was actually one of the
recurring checks and balances that have so far prevented women from
attaining equality as human beings.

The fact is, only after they won the vote was there any real pressure
for women to eschew the physical abundance that had been favored
since the beginning of time, and shrink down to the diminutive dimensions of powerless adolescents. Yet, the significance of this virtual
checkmate had been anticipated by visionary suffragist Lucy Stone way
back in 1855: "It is very little to me to have the right to vote, to my
own property, etcetera, if I may not keep my body, and its uses, in my
absolute right."

But women's bodies and dreams were still up for grabs after the
vote was won, as far as marketers were concerned. As long as they
kept bombarding consumers with the message that the true New
Woman had to be thin, antifat profiteers of all stripes could continue
making a buck. And advertisers had become a lot more adept at the
"art" of spinning such schemes than they were in, say, 1899, when the
cleverest concept the National Biscuit Company's agency could come
up with was a lame and unsubtle rechristening of the product as
"Uneeda Biscuit."

The Great Depression of the 1930s put a crimp in everyone's plans,
to put it blandly, and temporarily halted the mania to become skinny.
It wasn't simply that spending power plunged; for the majority of
women, the necessity of scrambling to get by left little time for pre-
occupation with artificial beauty standards. And it's easy to stay slender when you can't always afford enough to eat. Perhaps that explains
why, judging by the *Reader's Guide to Periodical Literature*, there

were seldom more than one or two magazine articles on the topic of slimness published per year during this period.*

Women's weight pretty much took care of itself during the Second World War as well, with the rationing of such fattening foods as meat, sugar, and butter, and, for many, through physical labor in the war industries. Other jobs vacated by men for the duration also sorely needed to be filled, and accordingly, women were admonished by a raft of magazine articles to break out of domestic confinement. Some of the most adamant of these were "Women Must Work, Not Only Weep" (*Social Welfare*, 1939), "The Hand That Rocks the Axis" (*Collier's*, 1942), "Key to Victory: Women in War Industries" (*Woman's Home Companion*, 1942), and "Women in Slacks Speed Plane Production" (*Reader's Digest*, 1942).

But as armistice approached, bringing with it the need to open up jobs for returning men, magazines began shoving women in the opposite direction. The social and psychological pressure for Rosie the Riveter to swap her dungarees for frilly dresses, and to otherwise "refeminize" herself, was swift and relentless. Certainly, much of this came from a genuine desire to restore family life. But the obligation for women to abruptly surrender the independence that had come with holding down jobs and managing on their own was rigidly reinforced by an onslaught of articles, short stories, and poems such as those in the January 1945 issue of *Ladies' Home Journal*.

Up front was the deceptively titled "The New Woman in the New America" by renowned columnist Dorothy Thompson. "The fact that in this war America has emerged as the premier world power," she wrote, "does not affect the cooking of breakfast, the dressing of children, the getting them off to school, and all the other routines of the domestic lives which are [women's] normal sphere."

Feature stories in this issue included "Diary of Domesticity," "A Mother-and-Daughter Room," "The Plus in Your Wardrobe," and "Where the Heart Is." The half-dozen fiction pieces focused on romance and had such titles as "You'll Marry Me at Noon." Among

---

*Even so, the savviest profiteers went right on developing diet pills such as amphetamines and testing other drugs, including digitalis and various sedatives, for use as weight loss aids.

the poems were "My Bride Forever," "Loving a Little Boy," and "None But the Lonely," the last a wing-clipping little tract which began: "None but the lonely hearted find / The road that leads to the highest place."

The "get thee homeward" theme was reinforced by many of the accompanying advertisements, especially those featuring teary-eyed women embracing returning soldiers and sailors. These ads included those for Community Silverplate (headlined "Back home forever"), Trushay lotion ("Part of your love story"), and Pond's hand cream ("It's easy to see why her tall blond Navy fiancé adores Patricia!"). In an ad for Lux soap headlined "I hurt Bob's pride by my dishpan hands," a chagrined woman extends her hand to an older man, who looks at it disapprovingly, while hubby Bob, wearing an army uniform, stands between them, scowling. Scott tissue's slogan was "He needs you more than ever in a war-changed world." And, tellingly, a packaged regimen called DuBarry Success Course featured a woman boasting "I lost 77 pounds in 6 months!"

Typically themed articles in other periodicals during this period included "Has Your Husband Come Home to the Right Woman?" (*Ladies' Home Journal*, 1945), "Should Women Return to the Home?" (*National Home*, 1945), "How Good a Mother Are You?" (*Hygeia*, 1945), "Have Babies While You're Young" (*Parents*, 1946), "The Best Place in the World" (*House Beautiful*, 1947), "Femininity Begins at Home" (*Ladies' Home Journal*, 1947), "Women Must Choose Privileges or Rights" (*Saturday Night*, 1947), "The Art of Staying at Home" (*Reader's Digest*, 1948), and "How to Get Whistled At" (*Collier's*, 1948).

Only a decade and a half earlier, the new possibilities epitomized by winning the vote had inspired numerous articles and short stories that "mirrored the yearning for identity and the sense of possibility that existed for women then," to quote what Betty Friedan would later write in *The Feminine Mystique*. This was startlingly evident even in material about traditional subjects such as "The New Era in Housework," published in the June 1929 issue of *Ladies' Home Journal*, which began: "There are at least six reasons why we have got this much nearer the workless home of the millennium. First, nowadays the female half of the race is taken as seriously—almost—

as the male half, and a good many first-rate brains are working on the problem."

Articles extolling loftier endeavors included "Women's Air Derby" (*Literary Digest*, 1929), "Opening the Pulpit to Women" (*Literary Digest*, 1929), "Women Winners of Foreign Trade" (*Business Week*, 1929), "How to Make Money in Wall Street" (*Woman's Home Companion*, 1930), "Our Glorious Sports Girls" (*Ladies' Home Journal*, 1930), "Power: United Forces of Women Can Provide Leadership" (*Ladies' Home Journal*, 1932), "She Got the Order: Only Saleswoman of Steel in the World" (*Collier's*, 1932), "I Can Count on Myself: Reflections of a Woman of 50" (*Scribner's*, 1933), "Women Intensify Their Flight to Peace" (*Literary Digest*, 1933), "Women's Orchestra Makes Its Debut" (*Commonweal*, 1935), "Brought Up to Do Something" (*Ladies' Home Journal*, 1935), "Women Microbe Hunters" (*Independent Woman*, 1936), and "What Ho! Able-Bodied Seawomen" (*Christian Science Monitor*, 1936).

After the end of the Second World War, however, the same magazines were, as Friedan phrased it, "crammed full of food, clothing, cosmetics, furniture, and the physical bodies of young women [with no trace of] the world of thought and ideas [or] the life of the mind and spirit." Now a cacophony of voices lectured women on how they should take care of their husbands, children, and homes, and what they should look like while doing so. In the January 1950 issue of *McCall's*, for example, the features included "You Too Can Make a Perfect Soufflé," "New Gas Ranges Fill the Bill," "Seven Steps to a Youthful Look," "Brush a Glow Into Your Skin," and "The Last Word in Coat Dresses." Eleanor Roosevelt's popular "My Day" column, which had addressed more ambitious queries not so long ago, now answered questions about turkey stuffing and meddling mothers-in-law.

And the celluloid dream machine kept pace, quickly replacing such inspirational prewar movies as *Hail the Woman* (1921), *Christopher Strong* (1933), *Design for Living* (1933), *Imitation of Life* (1934), *A Woman Rebels* (1936), *Dark Victory* (1939), and *Gone With the Wind* (1939), and motivational war-era movies like *Mrs. Miniver* (1942), *So Proudly We Hail* (1943), and *Tender Comrade* (1943), with such inanities as *The Bachelor and the Bobby-Soxer* (1947), *The Egg and I* (1947), *It Had to Be You* (1947), and *June Bride* (1948).

The Propaganda Machine Begins Going for the Burn

All in all, by the time the troops had marched home and women had been herded back to the kitchen, the real battles in what would eventually become the billion-dollar brainwash had begun in earnest, and articles about the necessity of being slim were becoming inescapable.

A golden opportunity for the antifat brigades to pounce presented itself in 1947, when Parisian designer Christian Dior decreed the "New Look." After two decades of relatively comfortable fashions, waists and midriffs were suddenly expected to squeeze into the tiny circumferences that best complemented Dior's voluminous new skirts. This was an especially tricky task for millions of mothers who'd grown a mite pudgy while giving birth to the first wave of baby boomers, and there was open rebellion for a short while (as we shall see in Chapter 9).

But women didn't really stand a chance of heading off an avalanche of admonitions to literally belittle themselves. Between 1949 and 1955, there were no fewer than sixty-five articles on slimming in major magazines, including "What Do They Say about You?" (*Woman's Home Companion*, 1949), "Thin Rats Bury the Fat Rats" (*Harper's*, 1949), "No Fads for Fatso" (*Newsweek*, 1950), "Hypnosis for Hips" (*American*, 1951), "Lucy Learns to Be Pretty" (*Woman's Home Companion*, 1951), "Talk Your Fat Away" (*Coronet*, 1951), "Hollywood's Favorite Sweat Shop" (*Collier's*, 1952), "How the Stars Stick to Their Diets" (*Woman's Home Companion*, 1952), "I Want to Have Babies and My Figure Too!" (*Ladies' Home Journal*, 1953), "Overweight, Our Biggest Health Menace" (*McCall's*, 1954), "Why Do People Eat Too Much?" (*Mademoiselle*, 1954), and "I Was a Hopeless Fatty, Now I'm a Model" (*Ladies' Home Journal*, 1955).

By 1948, the antifat profiteers had shifted their sights downward. A typical short story in *Seventeen* magazine, entitled "The Fattest Girl in the Class," followed the Cinderella-style formula that would thereafter be a staple of both fiction and nonfiction: girl gets fat, girl is ostracized, girl goes on diet, girl finds happiness. Other obvious examples of this phenomenon included "No Fatties in the Family" and "Don't Let Your Child Be a Fatty!" (both in *Ladies' Home Journal*, 1953).

Was it mere coincidence that all such women's magazines were then sailing on a bountiful sea of ads for the new consumer goods flooding into stores, including diet and beauty products? Not a chance, according to Earl Shorris, author of *A Nation of Salesmen: The Tyranny of the Market and the Subversion of Culture.* He argues that, by using teams of researchers, demographers, statisticians, psychologists, writers, editors, producers, and actors, marketing had become a science "that could determine the desires of the buyer . . . [by reaching] into the process of imagination to the very soul . . ."*

Working hand in glove in this process, of course, was the by now mighty public relations industry. When the century was still young, its pioneers, especially Edward Bernays and Walter Lippman, invented the classic techniques for what they called "manufacturing consent" that endure today. Creating and manipulating symbols was their primary method, writes Stuart Ewen in a sobering book called *PR! A Social History of Spin.* As far back as 1922, Ewen says, Lippman "saw the strategic employment of media images as the secret to modern power . . . [and that] the most compelling attributes of symbols . . . [is their] capacity to magnify emotion while undermining critical thought. . . ."

When the omnipotent new medium of television was added to the mix of "persuaders" who set their sights squarely on female consumers, Shorris says, it was strictly no contest. The consumerism-equals-happiness formula was drilled into viewers by the powerful sponsors of such early shows as *People Are Funny, I Remember Mama, The Arthur Godfrey Show, As the World Turns,* and *My Little Margie.* Result: "Before television, tastes changed slowly, but once life could itself be mediated every morning, noon, and night . . . ," says Shorris, "[marketing] had become one of the forces that determined the world."

The stifling effect of all this less-than-gentle persuasion on a captive audience of homebound women was not recognized until *The Feminine Mystique* made its explosive debut in 1963. But economist John Kenneth Galbraith has characterized the insidiousness of such pressure: "Behavior that is essential for economic reasons is transformed into a social virtue."

---

*Incidentally, the market research industry itself would grow to be a $2.5-billion-per-annum business by 1994.

Some of the quid pro quos were amazingly blatant. Preceding a March 1953 article in *Ladies' Home Journal* titled "I Was Too Fat to Have a Baby," for example, were no fewer than seven large ads related to the desirability of either looking slim or actually losing weight. These included one for Metropolitan Life Insurance that stated: "Overweight is our country's Number One health problem today"; another for Starlac nonfat dry milk; and four ads, each a half page or larger, for girdles with such evocative names as "Curvallure," "Secret Panel," "Profile," and the "Playtex Streamliner." This last ad featured actress Zsa Zsa Gabor posing in a strapless evening gown beside the words: "Hollywood stars and famous designers call Playtex the perfect girdle."

Just two pages after the feature article about the woman whose doctor allegedly told her that obesity prevented fertility was a big advertisement for Florida grapefruit that began, "Don't give an inch to your waistline." Four pages later, there was another diet story titled "How Florence Delfino Lost 25 Pounds as Millions Saw Her Do It on Television." Complete with "before" and "after" photos, this article was actually an "advertorial" for Knox Gelatine's "Eat-and-Reduce Plan," which promised that you could "Eat your fill and lose 2 to 5 pounds a week." Turn two more pages and there's a picture of a woman in high heels and a revealing shortie robe peering down at a scale and touting the advisability of "Start[ing] each day the Health-O-Meter way!"

This ad-heavy issue was typical of the women's magazines during these years, most of which ran stories nearly every month similar to the following, which appeared in *Ladies' Home Journal*: "I Lost Weight and Am Just Beginning to Live" (1952), "The Diet That Launched a New Life" (1953), and "A Size 18 in Red" (1952). This last one included a diet plan specially designed for "wistful Wilma," who was pictured gazing longingly at a bright red dress in size 12 even though she admitted that, unless she lost weight, her choices would be limited to "the size 18 racks of slenderizing blacks or subdued colors . . . to hide her superfluous padding."

By the end of the 1950s, the titles grew racier, and included: "From Hippo to Slimmo" (*Ladies' Home Journal*, 1957) and "From Fatso to Cool Cat" (*Parents*, 1958). "Reducing at $500 a Week" (*Reader's Digest*, 1958) was evidence of the growing popularity of expensive weight loss spas.

And, trumpeted the accompanying ads, galloping to the rescue of anyone who couldn't accomplish the feat on her own was a zealous cavalry brandishing an ever-expanding arsenal of weapons specifically designed for attacking avoirdupois. But, "as in all wars," said a *Newsweek* article on the phenomenon, "it is the arms makers who are growing fat. . . . [B]y promising to melt and float the fat right out of your body . . . several hundred firms each year float $100 million out of the pockets of some 5 million Americans determined to be thinner." Echoed *Reader's Digest* in 1959: "They Take Your Money, You Keep Your Weight." In fact, so many of the new weight loss products belonged in the snake oil category that, in 1957, the federal government appointed a congressional subcommittee to look into fraudulent reducing aids.

Why So Vulnerable?

If you're wondering how this lunacy could possibly have enticed so many millions of otherwise sensible people (an estimated 80–90 percent of whom were women), you're ready for another "if only." And it's a biggie. Overall, as I noted at the beginning of this chapter, grownups were still in style and in charge. So even if girls didn't want to look like their own mothers, they were still just as eager as their predecessors to grow up and enjoy the status of mature women.

Enter Twiggy, who symbolizes the factors that stopped that aspiration cold and pared the former variety of beauty standards down to a single icon for the first time in history. Her arrival was actually part of a mosaic of events, rightly dubbed a "youthquake," that happened when 78 million baby boomers hit their twenties. It should have been as predictable as it was inevitable that this demographic five-hundred-pound gorilla would soon be getting whatever it wanted. But, as you'll remember if you're in the vanguard of the boom, kids weren't yet taken seriously. You simply didn't count until you were an adult.

What helped overturn this verity fits the "if only" category. Who were the influential cultural arbiters up to this time? Before and during the Second World War, many were feisty women who were part of the first generation of females ever to not only vote, but also build professional careers. They were bold, visionary, and passionate about the potential of their gender. And they filled their magazines, movies, novels, and plays with messages that inspired women to be all that they could be.

But by now, these trailblazers had died, reached retirement age, or been finessed out the door to make way for men. And because of the paroxysms of the Depression and the Second World War, they never got a chance to pass the torch of independence on to younger women, who consequently remained oblivious to the struggle for female equality. So the media vehicles pitched at women limited their agendas to the pure domesticity that best served marketers. The initial result of the pioneers' disappearance was, as Friedan expressed it, that "the feminine mystique began to spread through the land, grafted onto old prejudices and comfortable conventions which so easily give the past a stranglehold on the future."

But it's the long-term effect that's crucial in the No Fat Chicks context. These perceptive, mature, *self-respecting* women, who had always fought for female equality, were simply not around to help mediate the havoc the youthquake was about to wreak, leaven the strictly male way of seeing things, or pass on to a new generation of women the principles of independence that had been struggled for so long, and won so recently.

If only the legacy of their perspective hadn't been dumped and forgotten like last year's skirt length, the march toward equality would, almost certainly, have continued, instead of languishing as little more than a faint memory until the late 1960s. And many aspects of modern life might be much healthier today. Near the top of a tantalizing list of might-have-beens is the probability that the billion-dollar brainwash could have been headed off or, at the very least, alleviated by sheer common sense.

Friedan has amply substantiated the disappearance of material about the achievements and aspirations of women, and other important general topics, by analyzing the July 1960 issue of *McCall's*. With a circulation of more than 5 million, this magazine was a giant voice, speaking at a terrifically interesting time in history. Yet a male editor told her, "You just can't write about ideas or broad issues of the day for women. . . . They aren't interested in politics, unless it's related to an immediate need in the home, like the price of coffee."

Consequently, that issue of *McCall's*, like its contemporary rivals, consisted of articles that, as Friedan expressed it, confined "woman's world . . . to her own body and beauty, the charming of men, the bearing of babies, and the physical care and serving of husband, children, and home."

Smack dab in the middle of the magazine was a glamorous four-page spread titled "Reduce the Way the Models Do." The article, which was highlighted on the magazine's cover, included a 1,200-calorie diet for "when, horror of horrors, a size 9 becomes a little snug." And sure enough, nearby was a half-page ad for a new liquid saccharine product called Sucaryl: "No thanks! No calories!" declares a slender woman in a striped bathing suit as she pours Sucaryl into a glass of iced tea.

Other magazines of this period were no less explicit about the primacy of domestic roles for women. Striking examples include dozens of features on food, fashion, beauty regimens, home decor, marital relationships, and the complicated factors involved in raising children. Accompanying these were a host of related advertisements, a sprinkling of which featured newly invented weight loss products.

The anything-but-coincidental juxtaposition of ads and articles conveying identical messages illustrates the state of the union between magazines and marketers by the early 1960s. To extend the connubial metaphor, there had been a complete reversal in who courted whom. Competition among women's magazines for revenue-producing ads had become so fierce that five such publications had already perished and several others were teetering on the brink. Thus, thanks to the law of supply and demand, the role of the marketer had changed from ardent suitor to domineering partner.

Actually, this was getting to be old news, even though the pretense of an impenetrable wall between the editorial and ad-sales departments persists today. The elaborately concealed truth is that the wall began crumbling as far back as 1899, when *Ladies' Home Journal* was brutally taught a prophetic lesson. After rejecting ads for dubious patent medicines, the magazine was hit with a boycott by all its other advertisers. By the following year, ads had surpassed circulation sales as the top income source for most newspapers.

Henceforth, the advertising tail would wag the editorial dog to such an extent that Chevrolet, for example, once censored the phrase "ford the river" from an episode of *Gunsmoke*; Ford in turn had the Chrysler building painted out of a backdrop depicting the New York skyline; Camel cigarettes banned all news footage showing No Smoking signs; and, in the most infamous such incident, the American Gas Association had the word "gas" cut out of the soundtrack of *Judgment at Nuremberg*.

The print media were no safer from the edicts of their advertisers. *McCall's*, for instance, devoted six pages in its March 1970 issue to a story praising the "glories of Haiti" and totally ignoring that country's appalling poverty and the brutal dictatorship of "Papa Doc" Duvalier. Why? Because its top advertiser, Sears Roebuck, told them to. Sears also flew in editors with suitcases full of the company's clothes to replace the locals' raggedy duds for the feature photographs.

Today this domination is (or should be) most obvious from the placement of big glossy ads on the right-hand pages of magazines and the relegation of editorial text to the more awkward left-hand pages, forcing frustrated readers to flip back and forth in pursuit of the articles for which they buy publications in the first place.

But this inconvenience is insignificant compared with the dire effects marketers have had on the volume and content of that wandering text. During the three decades since the 1960 issue of *McCall's* in which the Sucaryl ad was "editorially complemented" by a feature on dieting, advertising in women's magazines has reached such a saturation level that the average ratio is now 70 percent advertising to 30 percent editorial text. In a recent issue of *McCall's*, the content of only 49 out of a total of 184 pages was *not* ads or complementary copy.

What effect did this power shift have on consumers along the way? Says *Village Voice* columnist Leslie Savan, one of only a handful of journalists whose full-time job is ad watching, it was Pavlovian-style conditioning to get us to "pulse to the . . . one-two beat that moves most ads: problem/solution, old/new, Brand X/hero brand, desire/gratification." Watching and reading ads, she asserts in an intriguing book titled *The Sponsored Life*, gives us our "notions of what's desirable behavior, our lust for novelty, even our visions of the perfect love affair . . . [and] cultural forms that don't fit these patterns tend to fade away."

Après Twiggy, the Deluge

By the time Twiggy arrived in New York in 1967, the No Fat Chicks messages had been drummed in so thoroughly that dieting was already becoming a big business. Weight Watchers had enrolled nearly 500,000 members in its twenty-three franchises and spawned several imitators, all of which employed the peer-pressure techniques developed by company founder Jean Nidetch.

Within a year after Twiggy's debut, the editorial and advertising cheering sections at women's magazines had shifted into high gear and added exercising to their lists of must-do's. They were also pushing the concepts that being slim was a discipline women owed themselves, and that this was the only route to good health. *Mademoiselle*, for example, editorially lectured its readers in no uncertain terms: "Creampuffs, there's no escape. Whip yourself into super shape and stay that way."

Unsurprisingly, advertisers were kicking in some pretty big bucks by now. A saccharine company launched its "$500,000 SweetaStakes" with a full-page ad in *Ladies' Home Journal* and several other women's magazines in 1968. It featured rear views of four bikini-clad young women splashing into the surf atop a slogan that read, "If only we could send all you Sweeta Girls to Hawaii!" This ad appeared simultaneously with many others for such new diet products as Carnation's Slender shake, and chewy, chalky (as I recall) Ayds pseudo-candies, which sponsored full-page advertorials with such headlines as "Inside I Was Crying Until I Lost 105 Pounds." Even such older products as laxatives, fruit, and margarine got in on the act by positioning themselves as diet aids. A Fleischmann's ad showing a pajama-clad family doing sit-ups, for instance, appeared in a magazine near a cover story titled "How I Lost 80 Pounds in 19 Weeks by a Governor's Wife."

Two years after Twiggy's big PR bash, Weight Watchers' gross revenues had leapt to $5.5 million. And this was only a fraction of what *Business Week* estimated as the $200-million annual "waistline industry," which, the magazine stated, "was not only better than any previous year, but about $50 million over expectations." Included in the total were $50 million spent on exercise machines and gadgets and "multi-millions [more] on diet foods, diet advice, slimming sessions at expensive spas and at thousands of health clubs."

What was motivating so many people to spend so much money? More than any other single factor, it was the addition of morality to the weight loss imperative. Being slim was no longer just the best way to be attractive, or even healthy. Now it had become the same kind of fire-and-brimstone character issue that sexuality had been in Victorian times. Any woman who "let herself go" was now regarded as a sinner and therefore a fair target for disgust, ridicule, and ostracism.

That the simple desire for thinness had been transformed into a full-blown and far-reaching obsession by 1969 was evident in contemporary surveys among high school students indicating that the number of girls who considered themselves too fat had risen, in just three years, from 50 percent to 80 percent.

Before long, grade-school children would be expressing fears of becoming fat, and attempting to limit their food intake. By the 1990s, one in twelve girls would be vomiting and/or taking laxatives, according to a shocking book by Frances M. Berg called *Afraid To Eat*. This is scarcely surprising, considering that, among other brainwashing factors, they were specifically targeted by ads such as a TV spot for Fibre Trim. Two girls, who looked to be about seven or eight years old, spoke in French (with subtitles) about how slender one of their mothers was. "Aren't you jealous?" asked one. "Not as long as she tells me her secrets," replied the other.

Later, studies on even younger children would reveal that antifat prejudice was affecting kindergartners, who preferred dolls with such physical deformities as missing limbs and disfigured skin to those that were oversized. Why? Because, the children said, the chubby dolls were "ugly," "lazy," and "ate too much."

The psychological effects of this prejudice on overweight youngsters grew cruel enough to contribute to widespread depression and a teen suicide rate that has quadrupled during the past three decades. Bitter evidence of this was provided when a fifteen-year-old Florida boy named Brian Head brought a gun to school in 1994 after being taunted for years about being overweight. "I can't take it anymore," he said, and then shot himself to death in his classroom.

....

By 1970, an estimated 70 percent of American families were eating "low-cal" products. And serious money was also being spent at the doctor's office. In addition to handing out diet sheets and dashing off gimmicky best-sellers, physicians were by now prescribing some 10 billion amphetamines per year. Soon, thousands of them would add weight loss surgery to their range of services. For the sake of fairness, it should be noted that what led many medical professionals to ride the weight loss rollercoaster were reports from insurance companies that repeatedly ratcheted supposedly desirable weight levels downward.

Skip ahead two more years, to 1972. It was almost impossible for antifat profiteers not to make a bundle. Weight Watchers had spread to forty-nine American states, plus Canada, England, Australia, West Germany, the Philippines, and Israel; signed up more than 3 million people (a number that would triple over the next five years); and added a cookbook, a monthly magazine, and its own line of frozen dinners, soft drinks, and skimmed milk.

Among those who tried more drastic measures, the first generation of liquid-protein diets had resulted in at least three deaths. Temporarily banned in 1977, so-called protein-sparing fasts would make a big comeback after TV talk-show host Oprah Winfrey later used one to lose sixty-seven pounds (which rapidly found their way back during the following year).

With the 1981 publication of her *Workout Book*, Jane Fonda began creating a one-woman fitness empire that would soon extend to videotaped exercise lessons and many related products. Fonda also inspired a parade of other celebrities, who followed her lead with a stream of their own diet and fitness products. (By 1994, the total amount spent on exercise videos would exceed $285 million.)

In 1981 as well, *Business Week* estimated that "the diet-food business . . . represents . . . the fastest-growing segment of the food industry [with] 6.6% of all U.S. food sales [for a total of] $450 million . . . excluding diet soft drinks, which bring in an additional $400 million." Those figures, the magazine added, "may double, or even triple, within the next five years . . ."

What was even more significant in the No Fat Chicks context was that giant conglomerate companies, including Nestlé, Stouffer, and

H. J. Heinz (which bought Weight Watchers in 1980), had jumped into the diet industry and were by then "mounting intensive ad campaigns [to] garner shares of the lucrative market," according to *Business Week*.

By 1982, during the time I was struggling with my magazine weight loss series, the number of listings in the *Reader's Guide to Periodical Literature* regarding what was referred to by now as "dietmania" covered more than three pages and numbered more than 250 articles, mostly in women's magazines.

Later in the decade, liposuction would be imported from France, despite having caused the deaths of nine women. During its first six years here, at least twenty deaths were reported. Yet these casualties received so little publicity—in women's magazines or elsewhere—that the procedure quickly became the most frequently performed cosmetic surgery in history.

A ghastly counterpoint, although the cause-and-effect connection garnered little attention, was a growing number of articles about eating disorders. The first mention of anorexia nervosa was a small piece in *Science Digest* in 1970. Coverage leapt to dozens of articles every year over the next two decades, particularly in response to the 1983 death from anorexia of world-famous singer Karen Carpenter. Yet most stories about eating disorders lacked perspective and continuity and, as a result, were too haphazard to sound an alarm bell about an epidemic that would claim more than 11 million women and girls by the mid-1990s.

Strong-Arming the Little Ladies

Sey Chessler, who was editor-in-chief of *Redbook* from the 1960s to the 1980s, calls the relationship between marketers and publishers "a holdup." "Advertisers want to know two things," he told Gloria Steinem for her *Sex, Lies & Advertising* exposé: "What are you going to charge me? What else are you going to do for me?" Chessler added that he thought "advertisers do this to women's magazines especially, because of the general disrespect they have for women."

Steinem is one of only a few other editors to go public about the "what else?" pressures that are routinely exerted by marketers.* She cited some especially revealing examples from the years before *Ms.* finally booted advertisers out the door in 1990 and began subsisting solely on subscription and newsstand revenue. Clairol, for example, canceled its contract in retaliation for a brief news item in *Ms.* about the carcinogenic potential of hair dyes. And even when this was widely reported elsewhere and resulted in Clairol changing its formula, the company maintained it would never again advertise in *Ms.* Later, Revlon stomped off in anger over a story on events in the Soviet Union because the women featured on the cover weren't wearing makeup.

But nothing contributed more directly to the No Fat Chicks credo than the terms of *Ms.'s* contract with Maidenform lingerie, which presumably still apply to other magazines (I was unable to elicit confirmation or denial of this). "The very nature of the product [appeals] to the positive emotions of the reader/consumer," stated a standard ad contract. "Therefore, it is imperative that all editorial adjacencies reflect that same positive tone." What kind of articles did Maidenform explicitly exclude? "Illness, disillusionment, [and] *large size fashion*" (emphasis added).

An eye-popping article in the *Columbia Journalism Review* in 1990 not only amplified Chessler's and Steinem's contentions, but reported that newspapers, too, are now succumbing to similar squeeze plays. Even the once sacrosanct *New York Times* now runs "fluff" pieces about such exploitative beauty preparations as firming creams, complete with references to advertisers' products. These sorts of features, and especially those fairy tales for grown-ups—the "makeovers" that have become a perennial in women's magazines—are a "value-added" bonanza for marketers, all of whom are credited in the editorial text free of charge.

The *CJR* piece also spotlighted other methods by which marketers have helped create a hideously distorted and limited cultural climate

---

*Another is former *Vogue* editor Grace Mirabella, who revealed in her autobiography that her publishers, who had never before issued such an editorial edict, ordered her to virtually ignore the health risks of smoking. Why? Because tobacco companies were threatening to withdraw their multi-million-dollar annual advertising campaigns—not only from *Vogue*, but from all other Condé-Nast publications.

for women of all sizes. Because so many new magazines are flooding the market (580 in 1989 alone), the fight for pieces of the advertising pie became so ferocious that it led to a "revolution in marketing . . . [aimed at] specific groups of people with spending money." The result, says *CJR* writer Michael Hoyt, is that "many magazines are hatched more as marketing concepts than as editorial ideas . . ."

To see for yourself what Hoyt means, just check any newsstand for such obvious examples as *Fit, Shape* and *New Body*, plus such Frankensteinian slap-togethers as *Vie*. The July 1995 issue of this last publication sported Jane Fonda on the cover above the headline "Celebrity Diet Issue," and inside what its publisher described as "the health club industry's cutting-edge source for information and news" were ninety-six ad-packed pages that repeatedly touted fitness clubs and activities the magazine itself cosponsored, plus a cover line and no fewer than eleven big ads for its own powdered diet supplement.

As for the daily press, when the *Wall Street Journal's* G. Pascal Zachary investigated the increasingly incestuous relationship with marketers, he concluded that, "with newspapers facing tough times financially, [we] see an increase in [their] tendency . . . to cater to advertisers or pull their punches when it comes to criticizing advertisers in print."

Lest readers conclude that only the print media are dirty-dancing with advertisers, the *Journal's* Joanne Lipman reported that NBC TV recently reversed the horse-and-cart formula that had always prevailed in planning television shows and, instead, "solicited advertisers first— and promised to feature them in [a] program" that would be created later and custom-tailored to their wishes.

In addition, many movies are now similarly influenced by marketers, who contribute hugely to their budgets, not just in return for on-screen "product placements," but also for having their say about what movies get made and which actors are cast. McDonald's, for example, whose fatty foods virtually manufacture future customers for the antifat conglomerate, gave the producers of *Santa Claus—The Movie* $1 million in 1985, in part to fund the construction of a set resembling a glorified McDonald's restaurant, and spent $18 million more on advertising and cross-promotions. This was chump change by 1996, when the marketing budget for *Space Jam* soared to $70 million. The movie's inescapable blitz was aimed at attracting millions of children and sports fans and was considerably enhanced by the corporate interconnection achieved by recent mega-mergers between the *Time* empire, Warner Brothers, and ABC TV. Together, this megamonopoly controls toy stores, music, video, and CD-ROM companies, *Entertainment Weekly* magazine, *Sports Illustrated for Kids*, and TV cartoon shows.

What's the effect of these octopus-like tentacles all operating together? Says cultural commentator Naomi Klein, "they can now hijack our culture on every front and feed all the profits into the same pockets. . . . [Such] synergy has emerged as a means of controlling consumption so thoroughly that choice is practically taken out of the equation."

Just a Fairy Tale

The reason I've gone on at such length about the way marketers got their stranglehold on the mass media is to document the reality behind one of the most dangerous myths in our culture. We believe that those in the mass communications business—upon whom we are obliged to depend for news and information, and from whom we absorb ideas that help shape our lives—enjoy free speech. We are wrong. And it's costing us, big time.

The problem isn't just the deluge of diet-till-you-drop propaganda. It's also that economic self-interest excludes all contrarian balances to this point of view, while simultaneously limiting the space for coverage of other vital subjects. Put another way, as David Croteau and William Hoynes contend in *By Invitation Only: How the Media Limit Political Debate*: "The media may not directly influence what the public thinks, but it can have a profound effect on what the public thinks *about*" (emphasis added). And, adds journalist Mort Rosenblum in *Who Stole the News?*, to enhance profits, news organizations "favor impact over information and neglect . . . subtle but vital undercurrents . . . [that] like . . . deadly virus[es] gradually spread into a worldwide pandemic."

There could be no better example of this than the scant attention paid to the epidemic of potentially lethal eating disorders that now affect 50 times as many females as are, according to current estimates by the Centers for Disease Control and Prevention, those infected with AIDS.

Certainly there was a spate of scare stories about anorexia after Karen Carpenter died. But where is coverage of the fact that bulimia is now so prevalent among female college students (estimated at between 20 and 50 percent) that many dormitories have designated "vomiting bathrooms"? Or that "bulimia parties" are now a popular pastime on campus, during which female students—to relieve the pressure of habitual semistarvation—get together to pig out on junk food, and then to vomit?

And why wasn't writer Tina Gaudoin publicly rebuked for her irresponsible answer to charges that women's magazines exacerbate eating disorders by exclusively featuring super-thin and super-young models? "People were dieting long before newsstands were invented," she wrote in the July 1993 issue of *Harper's Bazaar*. Insisting that the skinniest models "eat like horses" and that "thin is their natural body type," Gaudoin added, in a facetious tone, that "the Greeks binged and purged, as did the Egyptians."

Quisling-style equivocations like this should alert us to the fact that freedom of the press has become just another of the fairy tales we're encouraged to believe. Yet another is that advertisements are, at worst, merely petty annoyances, no more life-threatening than gnats buzzing in our ears. But in terms of venerable fables, advertising is actually more akin to the king in *Rumpelstiltskin*, everlastingly holding consumers hostage so we can produce gold.

Or, phrased less fancifully by the authors of *By Invitation Only*: "Major advertisers, not individual readers or viewers, are the primary 'customers' for mass media organizations, who essentially 'sell' the audience to advertisers." *Ladies' Home Journal* provided dramatic proof of this contention when it placed the following ad in *Advertising Age* magazine:

> Hey Coke, want 17½ million very interested women to think Diet? Better than one out of three *Ladies' Home Journal* readers buy and drink diet soft drinks. . . . And, we give you all these trim, fit readers at the lowest, most efficient [cost]. . . . We give you a very healthy environment for your ads, too. With editorial that feeds the appetite for information . . . [and] with lively articles about staying in shape. . . .

What makes the whole situation even more insidious, charges investigative journalist Eric Clarke in a scorching book aptly titled *The Want Makers*, is that, by the time most Americans leave school, in which they spend an average of 11,000 hours, they will have watched up to 18,000 hours of TV, including 350,000 commercials. And "the more we are bombarded by advertising, the less we notice, and yet, almost certainly, the more we are affected."

Ironically, just three years after Twiggy's Manhattan triumph, she retired from modeling, saying she was sick of being "a thing, not a person." Her farewell statement might also have served as a fitting *finis* to the mania for extreme thinness she initiated, especially since she proceeded to gain twenty pounds so that she could become a credible actress.

But no one paid attention, and the fashion revolution Twiggy inspired rolled on without her. The swinging "unisex" styles kept zinging across the ocean from London's Carnaby Street to boutiques that sprouted up like psychedelic mushrooms from New York to Los Angeles. As youthful egalitarianism quickly supplanted high society's traditional influence on culture, miniskirts climbed higher and higher, bodices grew tighter and barer, bras were discarded, and girdles were out of the question. Soon there was nowhere to hide any body that was chunkier than those of the bony young "birds" who populated the coffee houses and discotheques, magazines, movies, and television.

If all this had been just a madcap fling for youngsters who were trying out their newly acquired wings, no permanent damage would have been done, and relative cultural sanity would have prevailed as usual. But the stylish image the youngest, slimmest women achieved so effortlessly was no longer just one of many available choices, depending on one's age, size, and circumstances.

This variety had always pertained in the past, as evidenced (for example) by the simultaneous screen popularity—just before the youthquake of the late 1960s—of zaftig movie stars like Marilyn Monroe, Elizabeth Taylor, and Sophia Loren; ethereal Audrey Hepburn; petite teenager Sandra Dee; and bony spinster types portrayed by Katharine Hepburn and Thelma Ritter. Concurrently, other prominent women were as variously sized as U.S. first ladies Mamie Eisenhower (stout) and Jacqueline Kennedy (svelte).

But after Twiggy, the standard of beauty crystallized into a single dominant body image mandated by those who, knowingly or unwittingly, were doing the bidding of marketers. So, even when hot pants, hip huggers, and go-go boots disappeared into history, just one body style remained entrenched as the only acceptable one to have.

The unprecedented power of this mandate is evident from the fact that every woman who aspired to stay in fashion had to obey the onerous new imperative. Standards became so extreme that the Duchess of Windsor's thirty-year-old aphorism "A woman can never be too thin or too rich" was taken literally for the first time. Even Jacqueline Kennedy, who *had* looked as narrow as an arrow throughout the Camelot years, now went on a diet to achieve the "right" look.

Meanwhile, those who couldn't clone the new image began what would become thirty years of alienation, marginalization, and exploitation. The devastating effects of this phenomenon on Fat Chicks like me, and the emotional distress that escalated into an epidemic of eating disorders among smaller women, are detailed throughout this book. For now, let's see how an already dire situation was exacerbated when women's bodies were taken hostage by what Susan Faludi has rightly dubbed the "backlash" against women's equality.

A Pig in a Poke

As the 1960s ended, feminists began achieving a modicum of credibility, despite stubbornly reactionary media obfuscation of their mission, typified by a statement in the July 1970 issue of *McCall's* calling "lib ladies . . . poor, strident, ridiculous, hung-up creatures."

Principles and aspirations that had been virtually forgotten in the half century since women won the vote began drifting back into national consciousness. Early consequences of this reawakening included the Women's Strike for Equality on August 26, 1970—the fiftieth anniversary of female suffrage—during which tens of thousands of women paraded in New York City, and many more refused to work, inside or outside their homes.

A few months earlier, more than two hundred feminist crusaders had stormed the headquarters of *Ladies' Home Journal*, occupying its office for eleven hours. Their demands were that the male editor-in-chief resign, and that the magazine allow them space in which to express their views. John Mack Carter kept his job, but printed eight pages on the women's liberation movement in *LHJ*'s August issue.

In time, the parallels between the 1920s and the 1970s became unmistakable and extended well beyond the proyouth transformation of music, movies, and other forms of popular culture—and the illusory fashion "liberation," once again represented by shorter skirts, scantier undergarments, and boyishly thin physiques.

What's far more significant is that the same Big Lie was trotted out by the powers-that-be in each era—namely, that society's blessing on these superficial changes somehow added up to the very freedom and empowerment women were demanding. This was howlingly untrue, as many cultural commentators, including Faludi, have pointed out. In *Backlash: The Undeclared War Against American Women*, she writes that "the feminist entreaty to follow one's own instincts became a merchandising appeal to obey the call of the market—an appeal that diluted and degraded women's quest for true self-determination."

Historian Roberta Pollack Seid translates the situation into the No Fat Chicks context in an equally powerful book titled *Never Too Thin: Why Women Are at War With Their Bodies*. "Ironically, as the role of women was redefined, theoretically empowering them, these very freedoms trammeled them even more with one enduring traditional pressure—the pressure to be thin."

The result? A cunning and hugely profitable smoke screen stalled the crucial advances that women were on the verge of achieving in the 1970s, exactly as its predecessor had done in the 1920s.

Zoom with me now back to some smoky boardroom in an advertising agency on Madison Avenue, circa 1968. The fellas slumped around a long, shiny table seem a little dejected. That's odd. Just yesterday, they'd been jubilantly slapping each other's backs as they pored over the latest stats from the demographics department.

Yum yum! Seventy-eight million baby boomers busting loose, feeling their oats, making their own money, just ripe for the plucking. And half of them are women—who'll buy anything that promises to make them beautiful. Here comes my cottage in the Hamptons. Hell, make it Palm Beach!

But the topic on today's agenda is bumming everybody out. Seems there are these broads writing books and making speeches and stomping around capital cities saying the end is nigh for every scheme and dream that worked so well in the past. This so-called New Woman is rising out of the rubble and rip-offs that lured her mother and grandmother into pursuing happiness by shopping their fool heads off. But the new chick says she's got no use for such gewgaws and fripperies. She's set her sights on—get this, Fred—saving the world. What the hell are we gonna do?

Fred takes a long pull on his five-dollar stogie, swings his Guccis up on the table, and chuckles. *Sit down, shut up, and stop getting your knickers in a twist, pal. The way out of this one is strictly a no-brainer. It worked before and it'll work again. Can't miss. All we gotta do is give her what she wants.*

Say what!!??

Ever heard of a little thing called a pig in a poke? That's when you say you're giving some stupid schnook what he asks for but you keep it wrapped up in what Southerners call a poke sack. Trust me, you tell him. You asked for a pig and that's what's you're getting. It's a wonderful pig. Probably the best in the world. You're lucky to get it. Off goes the schnook, happy as a clam. And by the time he finds out that what he really bought is a worthless alley cat, it's too late.

You say these broads want liberation? Well, we'll give it to 'em. Morning, noon, and night. They're demanding freedom and power? No problem. All we gotta do is keep coming up with the best damn poke sacks there's ever been.

Break out the brandy, boys, and let's get to it. The world is still our oyster. Always was, always will be.

Seen in retrospect, the marketing campaigns that responded most directly to what was then called "women's lib" were blatantly transparent. The most obnoxious example duplicated the 1920s scheme of equating smoking with freedom. It was, of course, "You've come a long way, baby," the ubiquitous slogan for Virginia Slims cigarettes. Virginia

Slims. Get it? This name proved so successful that the company later upped the ante by bringing out Virginia SuperSlims. Slogan: "More than just a sleek shape." Lately, as if to flaunt their success in snagging the fastest-growing sector of smokers in the country, the ad copy reads, "It's a woman thing."

Many similar ads, such as the grinning, pant-suited blonde striding aggressively on behalf of Charlie perfume, echoed the same strategy of appearing to salute women's new power while simultaneously implying that the truly savvy Ms. could score even bigger by buying their products. Except for this new "libber" twist, though, there wasn't anything novel about conning women into painting, powdering, perfuming, or clothing themselves. What apparently came into sharper focus among market researchers at this time—judging from the tenor of the contemporary articles and ads—was that the real gold to be mined was the body itself.

Not only was there a limit to how many new lipsticks, hair dyes, or dresses a woman was likely to buy in an average day, but a sharp downturn in both women's apparel sales and magazine subscriptions at this time evidently set off an alarm. It must have seemed just possible that the pesky feminists would rouse their sisters from their Rip Van Winkle snooze and foment widespread rejection of advertising's fundamental message—that women are not good enough as nature makes them.

But if the conviction could be implanted deeply enough, and reinforced strongly enough, that slender bodies actually symbolize the attaining of revolutionary goals, there'd be no end to the products that could be dreamed up and sold. Bodies as skinny as Twiggy's are not easy to attain or sustain. So if you're not born that way, you'll need a lot of "help." (Right, Fred?)

With that epiphany, the brainwashers kicked into overdrive. "Corporations saw . . . that there was gold in them thar thighs," writes media professor Susan J. Douglas in *Where the Girls Are: Growing Up Female With the Mass Media*, arguably the best of a slew of recent blow-the-lid-off books by a new generation of reform-minded women who are picking up where those 1920s pioneers were forced to leave off. Douglas argues that the mass media and the marketers who fund them did indeed co-opt the tenets of the women's liberation movement—and then sold those tenets back to us in a variety of artful disguises, as well as in such blatant rip-offs as that employed by Weight Watchers to introduce a new low-calorie bread: In a TV commercial and print ads, a trio of slim young women danced and sang ecstatically about the "taste of freedom."

As time wore on, more and more marketers of more and more weight loss products wised up to the "libber" strategy. The resulting ad campaigns ranged from pitches as obvious as Weight Watchers' to the far more subtle approach employed by peddlers of exercise equipment. These slick geniuses succeeded in almost subliminally equating physical fitness with political and economic power—even though what they're really selling is not genuine fitness, but simply personal narcissism.

Editorially complementing this type of advertising were scads of articles purportedly celebrating women's new clout. Seen through 1990s eyes, though, many of these were clumsily patronizing, and others were downright demeaning. The latter category included, in 1970 and 1971 alone, such outrageously sexist titles as "Women's Lib, the Tooth Fairy and Other Myths" (*Ladies' Home Journal*), "Pronoun Envy" (*Newsweek*), "Hey, Lady, What Are You Doing Here?" (*McCall's*), "Bride of Frankenstein" (in *Mademoiselle's* "Man Talk" column), and "It's Really the Men Who Need Liberating" (*Life*).

Marketers were generally much savvier than that. And their most ingenious lightbulb blinked on when they apparently realized that the way to *really* guarantee profits forevermore was to cast the standard of bodily perfection at lower and lower weights, until the "ideal" actually became unattainable for about 95 percent of female body types, henceforth they would simply sell the lie that this ideal *is* possible for those who purchase the right products.

And there were bonuses for those who swiped liberation's rhetoric, in that a woman didn't have to think of herself as a feminist to be hooked. If what she wanted was control of her professional career, this was soon so inextricably linked with controlling her size that salaries and opportunities for heavy women plummeted (as we shall see in Chapter 6), so she probably had to diet. If she wanted to look good to men, other women, or just to herself, as "good" was defined by the mass media, the standard was now so thin that she probably had to diet. If she wanted to fit into the most stylish clothing, which was rapidly being downsized (as discussed in Chapter 9), she probably had to diet. Even if all she wanted was to feel good about herself as an intelligent, responsible person who was maximizing her potential, she probably had to diet.

Achieving Orwellian Saturation

As with other propaganda campaigns throughout history, it wasn't long before what started out as an artificial, self-serving premise worked its way into the popular culture as conventional wisdom. A given. Just the way things are. Anything else becomes, at best, passé and, at worst, anathema.

Thus we ended up surrounded by inescapable reinforcement for the proposition that all women must be thin. It flickers before our eyes every waking moment in the estimated 1,500 images seen daily by Americans in print ads, TV programs and commercials, posters, store windows, billboards, movies, sports, magazine features, books, greeting cards, cartoons, and gag items.

Editors and writers developed amnesia about all but one body type. Casting directors narrowed their choices for plays, movies, and TV down to skinny and young. Comedians, both professional and amateur, easily grasped that, even amid growing "political correctness" regarding other minorities, it was still okay to make fun of fat people. Talk shows, if they addressed any facet of obesity at all, usually tried to outdo the competition by creating a circus freak-show atmosphere. And somebody somewhere let out a guffaw, slapped his knee, and came up with the moronic bumper-sticker that gave this book its name: NO FAT CHICKS!

As the iconographic power of slimness grew, even the venerable Coca-Cola bottle was streamlined to eradicate its classic hourglass shape. Later, the lady in the flowing robes who had graced every Columbia Pictures movie for seventy years would be whittled down. Later still, the Saks Fifth Avenue store mannequins that had been cast to resemble actress Grace Kelly's size 8 were replaced by size 4 clones of "superwaif" model Kate Moss.

In the magazines and on the fashion runways, the twirling girls grew thinner and younger by the year. In the movies, the actresses looked skinnier and skinnier. Watching television, we were trained by clever dialogue and canned laugh tracks to disregard the evidence before our eyes and accept that, in *The Mary Tyler Moore Show*, for example, the Rhoda character was too fat, while the Mary character, played by an actress whose diabetes kept her gaunt, was ideal—which, by then, was synonymous with normal.

As time went by, the beauty images women were trying so hard to imitate drifted even farther from reality. The weight of actresses, models, beauty pageant contestants, and even *Playboy* pinups plunged from a reasonable 8 percent below that of the average North American woman in the 1950s to 23 percent lower by 1988, and it has continued dropping ever since.

Meanwhile, real women were getting plumper with every technological advance that made physical labor obsolete, and with every new fat-laden prepared food that came on the market. By the early 1990s, the average weight and height of American women was about 140 pounds and 5 feet 4 inches.

But the brand of beauty they are now being being urged to attain is epitomized by the size-4 actresses on TV series like *Friends,* and by Kate Moss, who weighs in at a wispy 105 pounds. Although, at 5 feet 7 inches, Moss is only a few inches taller than the average woman, most of the other "supermodels"—who, by now, have achieved such primacy over actresses and other beauty icons that they've spawned their own dolls, magazine, and website—stand 5 feet 10 inches or taller.

The futility of trying to eradicate this wide a gulf should be obvious. Yet millions of women are obsessively attempting to do just that. All of which means that, as one leading physiological authority expressed it, "We now have cultural norms that are way out of sync with our biological heritage."

As if these factors aren't enough to put "the feminine esthetic at odds with femaleness in its natural state," as Susan Brownmiller phrases it in *Femininity* (another good contribution to setting the record straight), the beauty icons have become more and more bogus. Many (if not most) models undergo cosmetic surgery, usually to enlarge their breasts—thus manufacturing an anomalous body type virtually unknown in nature: buxom, but as skinny and narrow-hipped as a boy.

And the photographs that inundate the visual landscape are also "perfected" by increasingly sophisticated technology, which evolved from camera airbrushing to digital computer techniques. So, to quote a recent *New York Times* article, women now aspire "not to look like the great beauties of the generation but like an invented, manipulated, unattainable idea of beauty, a product of camera, darkroom, and computer technique."

This practice reached a peak of outrageousness (one hopes!) with the September 1994 cover of *Mirabella* magazine. The slender, unclad lass whom the editors touted as "personifying today's all-American beauty" wasn't even human. She was a "cyber chick" entirely concocted by a computer.

For real women, as we will see in the next chapter, the increasingly frantic dieting has turned out to be the equivalent of a forced march in the wrong direction. Food-deprived bodies fight back, exactly as they were programmed to do during cave-age famines, with the result that millions of women get fatter and fatter just by trying to get thinner and thinner. Like cars stuck in mud, the more they accelerate their efforts, the more hopelessly they are trapped.

Recently, a bold new brand of poke sacks was launched. Dieting is *out*, rejoiced a choir of familiar voices. "Fitness" is what the truly modern, truly intelligent woman owes herself. It's a fine concept. Too bad fitness, as defined by the chief profiteers, is just a euphemism for thinness. Too bad that yowling from the depths of this chic new poke is the same scrawny critter that's been trapped there for three decades, repeating the same old tune: "Buy, buy, buy!"

Bottom Line

Put plainly, what I call the billion-dollar brainwash was created by deliberately teaching women of all sizes to hate their bodies. And three Big Lies underpin the entire process: 1. that fatness is the worst cultural catastrophe possible for women; 2. that obesity must be voluntary because slenderness is available to all who pursue it with sufficient diligence and money; and 3. that the sole cause of all "excess" weight is therefore despicable self-indulgence.

Brainwashing the entire population to unquestioningly accept these lies paves the way for stigmatizing Fat Chicks—and guarantees that women of all sizes will frantically spend money on products that promise escape from that punishment. As the definition of the "ideal body" was set thinner and thinner, it literally became the impossible dream for the vast majority of women.

Am I saying the billion-dollar brainwash is really a conspiracy? Yes. Absolutely. The same kind of de facto, unorganized, indefinable conspiracy that kept women from voting for so long, and keeps us from achieving economic and political equality today. Can I prove it? Nope. All I can do is piece together the facts that *are* known, some for quite a while now, until the irrefutably horrifying puzzle portrait is revealed.

3

A Mountain of Mendacity

Never in the history of the whole hapless world has there been a hoax as lucrative as the billion-dollar brainwash. It is the closest thing to alchemy ever discovered—with a formula that turns fat into gold, and prejudice into profit. For marketers of a crammed cornucopia of weight loss products, services, books, videotapes, audiotapes, and clubs, it's like manufacturing your own customers. Better: It's like having them manufacture themselves and march to your door like a legion of zombies.

As P.R. practitioner H. A. Overstreet wrote way back in 1925 in *Influencing Human Behavior*, "[t]he secret of all true persuasion is to induce the person to persuade himself . . . [t]he rest will take care of itself." Or, as historian Carter G. Woodson once wrote about African Americans, "When you control a man's thinking, you do not have to worry about his actions. You do not have to tell him not to stand here or go yonder. He will find his 'proper place' and stay in it."

Nothing could exemplify this dynamic better than a trio of appalling attitudinal surveys. One, conducted by *Glamour* magazine in 1984, found that a huge majority of the 33,000 female respondents declared they would rather lose ten to fifteen pounds than achieve *any* other goal in life, despite the fact that only 25 percent were overweight and another 25 percent were underweight. Another, *Psychol-*

ogy Today's 1997 Body Image Survey, determined that 15 percent of
female respondents would willingly die five years younger if they
could achieve their "ideal" weight. And another poll, reported in
Newsweek in 1990, discovered that if informed in advance about a
fetus's predisposition to obesity, 11 percent of the surveyed couples
would opt to abort it.

By 1981, just a decade and a half after Twiggy's debut, the annual
take by the multifaceted weight loss industry had rocketed to an estimated $10 billion. That preposterous total would quintuple during the
following years. All in all, as of this writing, the latest figure being cited
by a credible source (*Psychology Today*) as the total annual spending
in the United States on weight loss products and services is $50 bil-
lion. That, according to *Money*, breaks down into an average of up to
$84 per pound *temporarily* lost, or about $500 per year per dieter.

And the true genius of this cavalcade of chicanery is that it pros-
pers despite achieving the exact opposite of what it promises. No one
even makes the connection between the deliberately induced delir-
ium and the fact that, during the three decades since Operation
Twiggy hit the Atlantic beachhead in 1967, most of us have become,
not thinner, but fatter.

So, by the desperate, gullible millions, we continue to scrape up
every dollar we can spare and trudge off to spend it on an array of
snake oil products and services that are almost as idiotic as the mythical fat-eating tapeworms women used to wish for, or the absurdities
Dave Barry dreamed up for one of his best humor columns ever. My
favorite among his imaginary devices: the "incredible Squee-Zer-Ciser
with the revolutionary new Iso-Flex Modular Torsion Units, which
look to the untrained eye like rubber bands."

Am I exaggerating? You decide, after checking out the following
outrageous examples of the innumerable diets, gimmicks, books, and
club techniques that began trickling onto the scene in the late 1950s,
revved up to warp speed a decade later, and roll on inexorably today
like a monstrous avalanche.

The first pebbles to roll down the molehill that became a mountain of
mendacity were laughable. These included such gadgets and gizmos as
a "magic couch" called the "Slendro Massager Table," on which clients

at some one hundred branches were gently jiggled during the mid-1950s for two dollars per session. Then there were Slim-Skins—rubber blow-up trousers attached to a vacuum cleaner so women could, according to an ad, "lose seven times faster." If that wasn't rapid enough, you could try mummy like body wraps soaked in an astringent that caused dehydration; or a rolling pin with suction cups; or a waist-constricting, heat-exhaustion-producing Astro-Trimmer sauna belt. All these products were, of course, "guaranteed" to make enormous amounts of flab disappear in incredibly short periods of time.

Later on, there were earrings to be massaged to thwart hunger pangs, though they usually produced only nausea; an electric "eating fork" with built-in red and green lights to tell you when to eat and when to stop; and a battery-operated device that yelled at you whenever you opened your refrigerator: "Are you eating again? Shame on you! No wonder you look the way you do." Later still, talking scales voiced similar insults, jaws were wired shut to prevent the eating of solid food, hypnotists "planted" relevant "post hypnotic suggestions," and subliminal-suggestion tapes played soothing music while, underneath, a faintly audible message nattered: "The fat is melting away."

Another range of choices—pills and potions—really took off after the introduction, in 1960, of a powdered mix called Metrecal (an abbreviation for "metered calories"). Just add water, stir, and consume instead of food. A few years later, there was liquid protein, a powder ostensibly consisting of just enough essential minerals to keep the body from looting lean muscle tissue. Four million people ended up trying it, according to *Newsweek*, despite the fifty-eight deaths related to its use that were investigated by the Centers for Disease Control and Prevention. Liquid protein's death-defying appeal was enhanced by the marketing flair of Dr. Robert Linn, who, in *The Last Chance Diet*, claimed that his own brand, Prolinn, had "the full pink tint of a Beaujolais." And Prolinn was labeled with an ingenious "cover-your-assets" statement that soon became the anthem of the entire weight loss industry: "The program cannot fail. Only you can fail."

If liquid protein didn't appeal, you could try human chorionic gonadotropin (HCG), composed in part of the urine of pregnant women, administered by expensive daily injections in the gluteus maximus, and supposed to dissolve fat. Did it work? Sure, as long as you ate only the accompanying daily 500 calories prescribed by doctors, who sometimes augmented HCG with amphetamines and/or diuretics to ensure convincing losses.

Yet another option for desperate dieters was delving into the many books that began jockeying for position in the health and self-help sections of bookstores. Actually, a few—such as *Pray Your Weight Away*, and *Help Lord—The Devil Wants Me Fat!*—even muscled their way onto the religion shelves. For those who stopped short of seeking divine intervention, there were tomes such as *Eat Fat and Grow Slim*, which was so ineffective that it quickly flopped. Yet, in 1961, an identical concept was published by Dr. Herman Taller as *Calories Don't Count*. Some 2 million copies were snapped up, even after the good doctor was convicted of conspiracy and mail fraud for touting and prescribing the (equally useless) safflower capsules he himself helped manufacture. Taller got away with a suspended sentence, a $7,000 fine, and a stern "tut-tut."

Dr. Atkins' Diet Revolution, published in 1972, trumpeted the sensational claim that the more fat one ate, the better. This preposterous notion so angered the American Medical Association that Atkins was called before a congressional committee in 1979. But, since his book continued to sell in the millions, he continued laughing his way to the bank and writing more best-sellers.

By 1983, there were 360 diet books in print. One of the most extreme of the gotta-have-a-gimmick biggies was *The Beverly Hills Diet*, in which author Judy Mazel recommended six weeks of eating practically nothing but fruit. Anticipating (correctly) that this would produce serious diarrhea, she wrote: "The more time you spend on the toilet, the better. On watermelon days especially, you can expect to urinate a lot. That's the idea."

If that wasn't horrid enough, you could try *Fasting as a Way of Life*, in which Dr. Allan Cott addressed the obvious problem of starvation by callously claiming that "any so-called hunger 'pangs' are simply normal gastric contractions or stomach spasms. They represent the sensation of hunger rather than true hunger."

By 1995, there were more than 700 weight-loss-related titles listed in *Books in Print*. Many were deemed, in a scathing article in *Con-*

sumer Reports, to be "nutritionally unsound and probably dangerous."
These included *The Complete Scarsdale Medical Diet, Beyond Pritikin,
Dr. Atkins' Diet Revolution, Fit for Life, Medical Makeover, The Fat
to Muscle Diet, The Diet-Type Weight-Loss Diet, Thin So Fast, Eat to
Succeed, The 35 Plus Diet, The 120-Year Diet, The Two-Day Diet, The
Hilton Head Metabolic Diet, The Beverly Hills Diet, The I Love New
York Diet, The Bloomingdale's Eat Healthy Diet, The Rice Diet Report,*
and *The Macrobiotic Diet.*

For those who preferred less solitary pursuits than reading, there
were soon thousands of fitness centers throughout the United States. So
many, in fact, that, by 1992, annual American revenues were estimated
at $8 billion. If fitness were, indeed, the real stock-in-trade of these
enterprises, their gargantuan profits might be justifiable. But truth would
prevail only if they changed their names to "thinning centers." Of course,
this prospect is as unlikely as the possibility that they'll begin revealing
their duplicitous techniques—which include persuading desperate people to sign contracts for expensive promises that cannot possibly come
true; routinely selling far more memberships than their spaces can
accommodate (deliberately depending on high attrition rates by discouraged members); and contributing to the dangerous myth that we cannot
be fit unless we incessantly "go for the burn" with complicated, exhausting workout routines that few of us can actually perform without the
"professional" help available only at their establishments. The implication
that there's no use in the rest of us even trying is unforgivable.

(By the way, if you ask a Fat Chick what it's like to don a leotard
and stroll into the average fitness center, she'll probably say she can't
remember, because it's been so long since she ventured into the Land
of the Snobbish, Sneering, Neon-Thonged Skeletons. Don't believe
her. The crushing embarrassment of being the fattest, most blatantly
stared-at and laughed-about person in the room never goes away.
What actually disappears, in this order, are a Fat Chick's money, her
confidence, and, finally, herself—never to return to the killing field.)

But the senior partners among the antifat profiteers were definitely
the weight loss clubs. Among the first in North America was TOPS
(Take Off Pounds Sensibly). There was a small membership fee, but
nothing to buy—only a swell chance to damage your self-esteem forever, because the club's modus operandi was based on shame.

Like those of its many successors—most notably Weight Watch-ers—TOPS sessions generally began with communal weigh-ins, before which most women jettisoned every scrap of clothing and jewelry pos-sible, right down to their wedding rings, to reduce the scale readings. This was followed by Alcoholics Anonymous style confessions, with each member guiltily citing dietary transgressions, or triumphantly recounting her successful abstention. The group would then boo or applaud accordingly, after which a (formerly fat) counselor would praise the losers and probe the rationalizations of the gainers. A typi-cal exchange (quoted in a contemporary publication) went as follows:

COUNSELOR: Why did you gain?

MEMBER: It was my birthday.

COUNSELOR: So what did you give yourself—a pot of fat?

In the early years, TOPS sessions were even crueler than that. Mem-bers who hadn't lost weight during the previous week were required to wear pig bibs, deposit fines in a piggy bank, and sing "the pig song," which went: "We are plump little pigs / Who eat too much / Fat, fat, fat / Fat and forlorn." For those who actually gained, rather than lost, it was even worse. They were tried in a "court of weights and mea-sures," and placed in the running to be crowned "Queen Pig."

Still Strictly Caveat Emptor

Think we're too sophisticated to fall for this kind of blatant bunkum today? Think again. Tapeworms are now being marketed on the Inter-net. Hypnosis is hotter than ever. "Smart" refrigerators, programmed to withhold snacks, are in development. The back pages of magazines are littered with ads for transparently dubious products such as Sauna Shorts, whose "thousands of thermo-active micropore cells . . . destroy deep fat particles"; and tiny Svelt-Patches guaranteed to restore "girl-ish figures" by "melt[ing] away body fat" when pasted on pertinent body parts.

Descendants of the good old "magic couch" still claim that passive "electro-muscular stimulation" will do the trick. And many current pitches are just as silly as those of the 1950s. Something called the Clinic-30 Program, for example, headlines its ads: "I Watched My Next

Door Neighbor Dispose of Half of Her Husband's Body . . . and I Didn't Call the Police."

Emotion-laden holidays, including Christmas, Mother's Day, and Valentine's Day, are being co-opted in ads for "the perfect presents": gift certificates for reducing centers and programs. Among other hot items are pills called "Jogging in a Jug" and a Japanese-manufactured seaweed soap that claims to lather fat away. There are also any number of "organic" creams that supposedly make unsightly "cellulite" vanish and dozens of stimulant-laced products sporting such aggressive names and slogans as Thera-Thin ("Neutralizes All the Calories in the Food You Eat!"), and Maxi-Slim ("The Ultimate Weapon Against Fat"). These are frequently packaged with testimonials purportedly from doctors and are freely available in pharmacies, supermarkets, convenience stores, and even gas stations.

And stacked in bookstores from coast to coast right now are such transparently suspicious best-sellers as *The Angels' Little Diet Book* (in which the author insists that heavenly helpers enabled her to lose 150 pounds), *Good-Bye Diet Demon, Lose Weight Religiously, 32 Days to a 32-Inch Waist, Sun Signs Dieting, Gone With the Fat,* and *The Love Hunger Weight-Loss Workbook.*

Less amusing examples of literary déjà vu are the reissues of both Atkins' and Mazel's books, and Barry Sears's sensationally popular bestseller *The Zone: A Dietary Road Map.* It's basically an arcane reworking of the theory that made Atkins so rich twenty-five years ago, i.e., that (to quote from *The Zone's* book flap) "eating fat doesn't make you fat." Sears also claims that readers can "reset [their] genetic code[s]." So it's out with low-fat carb consumption, and in with red meat, oils, such high-fat yummies as avocados, "Zone" shakes, and "BioZone" bars—all of which purportedly "neutralize" calories when eaten in a "scientifically designed" ratio. As for working out, Sears claims that "you can burn more fat watching TV than by exercising." By the way, he wants to make it perfectly clear that *The Zone* is not, repeat *not*, a diet. Capitalizing both on his book's current popularity among personal trainers in Lala Land and on the general notion that movie stars know the real "skinny," Sears recently opened a Zone Center in Hollywood. Price tag for the introductory package, including weigh-ins, meal plans, coaching sessions, and a starter pack of BioZone bars: five hundred dollars.

There's also nothing funny about the recent deluge of diet "wonder drugs," especially the potentially dangerous "fen-phen" combination described in Chapter 5. They're available only by medical prescription at the moment, and some weight loss centers, including Jenny Craig and Nutri/System, have doctors "on staff" for just this purpose. Others in the industry are lobbying hard for the demise of this protection, so they may add these medications to the list of expensive products they market to their millions of clients.

By far the most pervasive, and persuasive, of the would-be latter-day miracle workers are commercial diet programs such as Jenny Craig, Weight Watchers, Nutri/System, Diet Center, and Physicians Weight Loss Centers—all of which are excoriated by the authors of a powerful exposé called *Feeding on Dreams: Why America's Diet Industry Doesn't Work*. What these "unregulated, unqualified, and unlikely to change" companies really sell, say authors Diane Epstein and Kathleen Thompson, are hope and instant gratification—"no work, no muss, no fuss. Just walk through our doors . . . and we'll turn your world right side up and put a smile on your face."

How do the programs lure so many millions of customers despite their, by now, well-publicized failure rates of 95 to 98 percent? Epstein knows all too well. She worked for twenty years at weight loss companies she now declines to name, for fear of being sued. The trickery begins, she says, with advertisements heralding low, no-strings-attached, introductory offers. Especially ubiquitous after New Year's to capitalize on postholiday guilt,* these are usually just classic "bait-and-switch" techniques designed to lure customers into showing up, ostensibly for individualized free consultations—but actually to be bombarded with high-pressure sales pitches. Epstein says that any counselor caught deviating from her company's telephone script by quoting the real fees is automatically fired.

So what are the actual costs, what do they buy, and what happens when an unsuspecting woman walks in the door? It varies, but not by

*In January 1994, for example, there was a "$50 million spending spree" on TV, print, and radio advertising for weight loss products, according to *Marketing* magazine. This was, of course, complemented by a flood of editorial stories about how to lose the pounds supposedly packed on during holiday feasting.

much. To begin with, there will almost certainly be a warm welcome from attractive, slender, female "counselors." These women may or may not be wearing crisp white lab coats that suggest medical qualifications few of them actually possess. They will undoubtedly weigh the customer and measure her pertinent girth—although the resulting numbers may be artificially increased by a deliberately loose measuring tape or the secret depressing of the scale by a sly finger. In any case, the numeric results will be dutifully recorded in a "personalized" chart. The friendly staffers may or may not take the customer's blood pressure and ask for details about her health history. All smiles and solicitousness, they will wax poetic about their dedication to providing their clients with supportive counsel, nutritional education, and behavior-modification techniques.

This is window dressing. The real function of these "counselors" is to reel in the fish their companies' ads hook. To that end, they will probe their customer's motivation for wanting to lose weight. Is "that special man" less attentive these days? Are the kids reluctant to bring friends home? Is a deserved promotion proving elusive? Has appearing in a swimsuit become embarrassing? Not to worry. That's exactly what the counselors are there to help with.

Oh no it isn't. Their real function is to "upsell" so effectively that what starts out as a "limited-time offer" freebie, or possibly a $19.95 special, or perhaps a dollar-a-pound deal, metamorphoses into a commitment of hundreds, and even thousands, of dollars.

How? In most cases, the introductory fee will cover only the first four weeks. Remaining in the program longer may cost as much as $80 per week, although this total is frequently veiled by incremental packages, billed seductively as "super-savers," or some such. How many weeks will you be advised to sign up for? That depends on how many pounds there are between you and your "goal weight." Who sets this? Not the customer, but the counselor, whose trusty computer has been programmed to recommend Twiggyesque weight levels.

The basic process is illustrated by an astounding, but typical, example cited in *Feeding on Dreams*. A woman visits a diet center with the notion of paying $19.95 to lose 10 pounds. No, no, insists the computer; you should really lose 20 pounds, at the eminently safe rate of 2 pounds per week. Now, says the counselor, we'll need your check for the registration fee (which ranges from $52 to $79, depending on location), and, after that, the weekly fee ($37 to $53). And, since retaining weight loss is such a chore, we strongly recommend that you enroll in our maintenance program, which lasts a whole year and costs only $110. Plus, you can't go wrong with one of our motivational tapes, audio or video, for only about $90.

All of which adds up to a total tab of between $642 and $829, right? Not after another quick upsell, it doesn't. The dieter's got to eat *something* for those ten weeks, but counting calories and fat grams is so tedious and confusing. Far better to buy the company's very own packaged foods and drinks (which are actually mandatory at some centers, including Jenny Craig). What's the tab? About $70 to $80 per week, which brings the total up to between $1,342 and $1,629—a far cry from $19.95. And what will these big bucks buy? Usually just a quick weekly weigh-in, a few (scripted) minutes of a counselor's time, and yet another shopping session for packaged foods.

Is anyone ever turned away because she's not heavy enough? Most diet centers say yes, but admit that they keep no records to back up the contention. Which is why an enterprising television reporter, who weighs only 109 pounds, recently hid a camera under her size-XS sweatshirt and ventured into a Jenny Craig outlet. Would they help her achieve an ideal figure? asked Karen McCairley, of Toronto's Global TV news team. Absolutely, she was told. And all it will take is a registration fee of $170, and a six-month stint at $100 per week, including meals.

But let's say you're too intelligent to get sucked into this expensive quicksand. You've decided to stick with good old feet-on-the-ground Weight Watchers. No phony lab coats, no quickie medical exams, no money up front, no year-long commitments, and membership fees of only a reasonable $12 a week. Time was, your logic would have been impeccable. But, after the humongous H. J. Heinz Company bought Weight Watchers in 1980, the top brass suddenly saw that membership fees were nothing but small potatoes (pun intended). Since then, the once humble support group has been transformed into a virtual supermarket of more than 250 food products bearing the WW label. From breakfast, to lunch, to dinner, with snacks galore in between, there are multiple choices of foods and drinks. They're now available in food stores, corner convenience marts, and at Weight Watchers' own retail shops, which recently began appearing in cities all over the continent.

What's a typical WW tab these days? Repeating the example of a woman who sets out to lose 20 pounds in ten weeks, we would begin with a registration fee of approximately $39, followed by $12 per week for the remaining nine weeks. Meals, on WW's popular Personal Cuisine plan, will run about $70 per week for the first three weeks. That goes down to about $50 per week for the final seven weeks, because members are advised to begin resuming "normal" eating for two meals a day. Total: $707. If, that is, she doesn't snap up any of the cute items on display at the WW shops and in advertisements in its monthly magazine, which range from gourmet coffee to tote bags, T-shirts, barbells, and cookbooks.

Mind you, she could take a more economical approach by reading one of WW's lavish brochures (sample headline: "As sure as the sun comes up, you *will* lose weight on Superstart! Guaranteed.") She might start by snipping out the many coupons that are strewn throughout a typical brochure's twelve glossy pages. And she could even drop her registration fee altogether by persuading a friend to sign up. Too busy, or located too remotely, to make it to a WW class or shop? No problem. There's a handy 800 number. Just ask for a "Weight Watchers at Home" kit (all major credit cards accepted).

Is my use of the term "chicanery" at the outset of this chapter starting to seem more charitable than churlish? How about if I toss in a scandal that recently made headlines in England after governmental weights-and-measures inspectors raided a popular chain of reducing centers, where the scales had been rigged to fool customers into believing they were losing weight? Or the fact that members of some fitness clubs in this country report that scales are weighted the opposite way, presumably to reinforce their motivation to reduce?

Or that no commercial weight loss center maintains records of, let alone announces, its success rate—which they'd surely be shouting from the rooftops if their methods actually worked.

Or that some of these organizations are already planning for the inevitable (one hopes!) day when consumers wise up en masse to their staggeringly high failure rates. How? By giving up on the truly obese, and instead targeting a more manageable market: the millions who think they "should" lose ten to thirty pounds, and do so—over and over again.

Or we could discuss the strategy by which a company doesn't even have to run a club, or operate a center, to get in on the action. If the billion-dollar brainwash hadn't turned millions of us into desperate fools, would a company like Nestlé think it was worthwhile to launch a single new meal-replacement beverage—Ultra Slim-Fast—with a $77.6 million advertising splurge? Would Weight Watchers follow suit with an annual ad budget of $40 million, or Jenny Craig top even that with an annual $50 million binge, if they *weren't* convinced we're now so crazed we'll buy anything that promises weight loss—and spend any amount on it? "What have you got to lose?" Jenny Craig asks in most of its sales pitches, and in the title of one of the founder's best-selling books. To which, I believe, we should all be replying: What indeed?

Jenny probably won't answer the question. But, incredible as it seems, a group of scientists did so fifty-three years ago—when, to their surprise, they learned exactly what's at stake for people who embark on deprivation diets.

To understand the basis for their conclusions, let's trek back to prehistory, when cave dwellers existed in feast-or-famine conditions. One week, they'd be gorging on woolly mammoth (or whatever), and the next, they'd be starving. The bodies of those who survived became very efficient at storing and retaining fuel—in the form of fat—to tide them over until their next feast.

Many millennia later, thanks to the legacy of natural selection, we're still programmed for survival in exactly the same way. Which means that whenever we drastically limit our food intake, the technique that worked so well during cave-age famines kicks in and holds on tight to the very fat we're trying to get rid of. How? First, the body uses the other available elements of water and muscle, and only when those are drastically depleted does it dip into its warehouse of fat for fuel. Then it cleverly slows down the metabolic rate at which activity burns off the remaining fat.

As if this fail-safe mechanism weren't enough to scuttle even the most determined reducing effort, what happens when we stop dieting is even worse. As we resume normal eating, the body stays on "famine alert" by keeping our metabolic rate so sluggish that exercise and other activities burn off fewer calories than they would if we weighed the identical amount but had never dieted. And lean muscle tissue is no longer available to burn food energy efficiently because it was jettisoned to keep us alive. So eating the same amount that kept one's weight steady before the diet will now result in a gain.

And, as proven by several studies (most notably that done at Rockefeller University), each time we repeat the process, we incrementally boost our "set-point" (which is the biologically determined natural weight level our bodies strive to maintain). So, no matter how low our postdiet weight, even moderate eating packs the original pounds back on, plus more to boot, because the body is trying—even harder than before—to store up fuel.

Multiply all this by the number of times a woman has dieted, and you'll see the ultimate results of what I've dubbed the "Cro-Magnon Catch-22." It's called the yo-yo syndrome, but that's not really accurate because a yo-yo stays the same size during its travels. But a body that endures repeated deprivations gets bigger, and more metabolically inert, with every bounce. Yet the sad irony is that most people, including Fat Chicks themselves, think they stay heavy because they aren't trying hard enough.

This reality is, of course, the exact opposite of what we have been conditioned to believe. To counteract this smoke screen of misinformation, we have only to consider a groundbreaking scientific experiment that should convince even the stubbornest naysayer that the body's imperatives are implacable, and that food deprivation has such a powerful effect on the mind and body that depression and bingeing are the inevitable consequences.

It began three months before I was born, and I can't help thinking that my life, and those of millions of others, might have been completely different if its findings had been embraced by the medical community. In November 1944, thirty-six conscientious objectors to the Second World War volunteered for a project at the University of Minnesota which remains the most comprehensive examination of semi-starvation ever undertaken. All the participants were healthy young men of average height and weight, and they were reportedly enthusiastic about the exercise, whose purpose was to learn how best to restore the health of people who were starving in the war zones.

For the first three months, the volunteers ate well-balanced meals, totaling 3,500 calories per day, and everything was peachy. Then their rations, although still sufficiently nutritious, were cut in half for three months. All hell broke loose. The formerly cheerful men became irritable, lethargic, apathetic, food-obsessed, and so argumentative that their regular group meetings had to be canceled. Two of the volunteers had emotional breakdowns and had to leave the project, while a third chopped off the tip of his finger so that he would be allowed to drop out. Even though the men were not starving, according to medical criteria, they were obsessed with food and barely functional. As Dr. William Bennett and cowriter Joel Gurin describe the situation in *The Dieter's Dilemma*: "The only clear fact was that prolonged deprivation of food was sufficient to produce extreme misery."

The final segment of the experiment was to have been a three-month period during which normal eating would be gradually reintroduced. But it didn't work out that way. Bennett and Gurin quote the original report: "The urgent desire for dietary freedom expressed by the men was extreme; postponement for [even] another week could have produced severe emotional crises and possibly open rebellion."

This despite the fact that the volunteers' daily intake was by then 4,000 calories—500 more than they had started with! And the men were still ravenous when they got together for a farewell banquet four months after the program ended. "The overriding sense of hunger these men felt was not appeased even by a large daily excess of food," say Bennett and Gurin. "Thus, even though their bodies were taking in considerable food energy, the profound psychological alteration that semi-starvation had produced remained with them."

Keeping this fascinating tale in mind, ask yourself how many diets you've ever been on that allowed you to eat as many calories—i.e., 1,750—as these guys nearly went bonkers on? In fact, how many of us eat that much even when we're not dieting? Today this kind of deprivation is just considered normal for women.

Actually, for many dieters, it's even worse. As Naomi Wolf reminds us in *The Beauty Myth*, "At Treblinka [concentration camp], 900 calories was scientifically determined to be the minimum necessary to sustain human functioning." Yet some of the most popular diets of our time allow little more than half that amount.

When I fasted for five excruciating months, consuming only water and a liquid protein called Optifast, my daily intake was a scant 600 calories. Did I flip out? Not quite. I banished every food from my kitchen except a jar of mustard. And late at night, when I couldn't sleep because of hunger pangs, I found it comforting to dip my finger in the mustard and slowly lick it off. Pathetic, yes. But at least I didn't chop my finger off, like that poor conscientious objector, who was taking in nearly three times as many calories as I was, and wasn't holding down a full-time job, let alone suffering psychological stress from a lifetime of feeling ashamed.

It has taken nearly half a century for medical scientists to even begin catching up with their collegial ancestors. In fact, only in the past few years have researchers managed to shelve the automatic assumption that all obesity is caused by the sins of gluttony and sloth. Their subsequent discoveries—particularly the isolation of the "ob" gene that apparently regulates fatness in the human body—are extremely promising. Similarly, the recently announced theory that fitness can result from, not mandatory hours of exhausting daily workouts, but as little as thirty minutes per day of such sensible, practical exercise methods as walking, is a tremendous boon.

Needless to say, however, the antifat profiteers are not taking all this lying down. Their mega-fortune is threatened as never before by the prospect that the conundrum of obesity may soon be solved, and ultimately redressed with responsible medical intervention and self-managed weight control regimens—instead of expensive, ludicrous, counterproductive snake oil. The industry's collective back is not to the wall yet, but it's abundantly evident that its members are striving mightily to preserve the status quo.

So, for the foreseeable future, our perspective on the billion-dollar brainwash must continue to be guided by this nutshell analogy: Suppose that 95 percent of all the computers on the market either didn't work from the get-go or crashed later on. Whom would we blame? The designers of the computers? The manufacturers? The retailers who sell them? The advertisers who tout them as magical marvels?

The repair technicians who, when asked for help, just shrug their shoulders? How about the salespeople—in the stores and in the mass media—whose persuasive powers convince everyone that life without computers isn't worth living?

Answer: None of the above, because denouncing any of these factions could lead to financial disaster. The only way to protect profits is to blame the poor schnooks who buy the computers.

So we tell everyone it's the schnooks' fault the computers don't work. And that, truth be told, they're really just a bunch of hopeless whiners anyway. Then we repeat, repeat, repeat this message until everybody believes it without question, laughs out loud at the schnooks, and takes every opportunity to accuse them of screwing up their own computers because they're lazy, stupid, and shiftless. Then we pass the belief on to children as accepted wisdom.

Result? Crazed by guilt and bewilderment, and desperately seeking a way to escape all the punishment, the schnooks have only one option: Buy another computer. And when that one doesn't work, buy another. And then another . . .

Substitute weight loss schemes for computers, Fat Chicks for schnooks, doctors for technicians, and antifat profiteers for salespeople, and you'll see the whole mendacious mess for what it is: a colossal con game.

4

Crazy or What?

....

How does it feel to belong to the only group in contemporary society that's still considered fair game for prejudice, exploitation, and outright cruelty? What's it like to live exempt from the laws and standards of communal behavior that now protect every other minority? It's so psychologically painful that, whatever their weight, virtually all American women now fear this fate.

SEVEN A.M.: "And finally, folks, this just in. According to a recent poll, 11 percent of those surveyed say they'd choose abortion rather than have babies who were prone to obesity. There ya go. Better dead than fed."

"Jeez"—the disc jockey chortles to the news guy—"if only Roseanne's mom and dad had thought that way, we wouldn't have to watch her waddle to the fridge for another tub of that loose meat!"

"Yeah," cracks the sports announcer, "whadja think's in that stuff anyway? A jillion calories of ugly?"

All three laugh as, somewhere in the listening area, a plump hand reaches out and switches off the radio. The woman rises and pads down the hall, showers, and does her makeup and hair, avoiding all but superficial glances in the mirror. Better not to see what even she's been brainwashed into loathing.

She casts a wary eye at the scale, but resists the compulsion to step on it. For once, she'll stick to her vow not to begin every day with a guilty verdict from a hanging judge.

To her closet. Hot weather is forecast, but she chooses something that conceals the maximum amount of detested flesh. Snips out the double-digit size labels that testify against her even though the chance of anyone seeing them is zip. Curses the compromises she's been forced to make in style, color, and price. You take what you can get.

Rouses and feeds the children and hustles them out the door. But not before battling another refusal to eat from her slender adolescent daughter. "I'm getting as, uh . . . as big as a pig, Mom." And not before being reminded that even her children think the word "fat" is an obscenity.

Drops the youngsters far enough from the schoolyard so other kids won't get the opportunity to embarrass them with nasty remarks about their mother.

Drives to her fitness center, where she's blatantly stared at and whispered about from the time she hits the locker room to the moment she heads back to her car. Oh well, she consoles herself for the umpteenth time, at least it's not as bad as her old club, which forced members to swim underwater to the pool it shared with an adjoining hotel, and then to remain submerged to the neck to spare hotel guests the sight of excess avoirdupois.

Hits the highway and tries to ignore the usual morons puffing out their cheeks and gesturing at her from other cars. Winces at the irony of a Joni Mitchell song on the radio: *You snipe so steady / You snub so snide*.

Rushes to a doctor's appointment. Tries not to bite the doctor's head off when he bluntly implies that her sore throat is somehow the result of obesity. Decides not to ask him about a suspicious lump because that would mean undressing and being seen and touched by someone she obviously repels. Bad enough that he seemed annoyed at having to hunt for a large-size blood pressure cuff.

To work. Not a great job, and certainly an unfairly meager salary. But the only one she could get after being fired under suspicious circumstances. But two lawyers said she'd be a fool to sue. Her credentials landed her interviews for better jobs than this one, but her appearance got her crossed off the candidates' lists, at first glance.

So what if her coworkers here exclude and avoid her as if they thought obesity was a communicable disease? So what if almost no one seems to see or hear her in meetings? So what if she has to remember not to turn so quickly that she catches colleagues gauging her girth? So what if the occasional wag anonymously sends her the latest Ann Landers column complaining that overweight people take up too much room on public transportation?

So what? It's a paycheck, and she needs it more than ever since her husband made good on his threat to walk out if she didn't get back to what she weighed when she was twenty. Funny how he forgets that, back then, he said she was too skinny.

ONE P.M.: Today she's got a rare lunch date with a friend. So at least the gang at the company cafeteria won't be checking out her tray. And it isn't as embarrassing when she doesn't actually know the diners who peer disapprovingly over their menus and glare when she squeezes between their tables.

FIVE P.M.: To group therapy. "What can I do about my constant anger, doctor?" "Why can't they understand that just because we haven't succeeded doesn't mean we haven't tried our hearts out?" "Why don't they just tell us not to breathe and be done with it?"

SIX P.M.: Her hair is sorely in need of a trim, but she's sick of having everyone stare when she refuses to change into a smock that's way too small. And she's tired of wondering whether the stylist will obey her instructions or just butcher her hair with a rush job, because who cares what a Fat Chick looks like?

To the mall. Total immersion in the unkindness of strangers. And she's in such a hurry today she can't manage the mincing, controlled steps that minimize both her jiggling and the corresponding catcalls.

To the bookshop. Past all the shrieking magazines. "Downsize Those Thighs." "Firm Your Butt Fast!" Tries to ignore the "joke" greeting cards featuring naked three-hundred-pound women eating cake. Pretends she hasn't heard a couple of jerks paraphrasing the title of a recent best-seller for her benefit: "Should be *Women Who* Waddle *With the Wolves*."

A quick dart into a department store, then a long hike down to the large-size women's clothing department, somewhere between the gerbils and the lawn mowers. What a surprise—apologetic polyester pup tents are still in this season. With ruffles.

Tries on a few things. Snarls to the unsympathetic mirror that designers obviously think chubby women have Arnold Schwarzenegger's shoulders, King Kong's arms, and Phyllis Diller's taste. Buys an unreasonable facsimile of what she needs. Tucks the telltale shopping bag inside the bookstore sack for camouflage.

Hurries past window after window of attractive, appropriate clothes. Remembers that not so long ago, their regular sizes ran big enough to fit her. Now they stop at 14 or smaller. But, hey, that chic blue tunic looks kind of roomy. Maybe she'll . . . No, better not risk it. Last time she ventured in there, a clerk stomped clear across the store to snarl, "We wouldn't have anything for you!"

To the supermarket. As usual, muffled snickers pursue her all the way to the checkout. As usual, everyone stares at what she's tossing in her cart. Band-Aids, broccoli, or butterscotch cookies, it doesn't matter. They all draw the same disdain. At least this time nobody reaches in, snatches out something they think is fattening, and tells her—"for her own good"—that she shouldn't buy it.

Home. Quickly scans the mail. Finds another anonymous letter telling her to "do something" about her weight because "people are talking." The first time she got one, she believed it was on the level, and felt humiliated for days. Now she knows the poison pen letters are actually a marketing ploy by a nearby weight loss center.

Prepares a nutritious dinner for the kids and low-fat frozen goo for herself. She eats four bites and has to vomit, thanks to a stomach-stapling operation that left only her bank balance slimmer. "Why did I mutilate myself like that?" she wonders, for the zillionth time. Then she remembers how desperately hopeful she was back when she still believed her naturally zaftig physique could be perma-shrunk down to "the ideal."

Decides to cut her night class. Can't face the professor making her the butt of yet another "friendly" jest. Decides not to jog or ride her bike, even though she'd love to work off some tension. Neighborhood teens have taken to oinking and mooing whenever she passes by.

Phone rings. A reasonably nice guy, asking for a date. She puts him off. Nonstop rejection makes it tough to trust even someone who seems to appreciate her. Besides, nowadays she flinches if anyone so much as pats her fleshy arms.

Quiet at last. Her stomach growls to protest the lost dinner, so she peers into the fridge and cupboards. Then decides that hunger pangs will be easier to cope with than guilt feelings. Settles for yet another of the eight glasses of water her nutritionist insists she gag down every day.

Sinks exhaustedly onto the sofa and skims a magazine article about being overweight. Stops when she reads, "The thought of anyone parading nude in front of a mirror at 190 pounds literally makes me gag."

Peruses a psychological self-help book someone recommended, but slams it shut when the author states: "I have always been repelled by fat women. . . . How dare they impose that body on the rest of us?"

Scans the local paper. In the news section: "Eating disorders triple in last decade." On the editorial page: Yet another cartoon using fat to symbolize evil. In the TV listings: Tomorrow's talk-show topics—fat, fat, fat. In the companion ads: Wanted—slim, slim, slim. In the Business section: "Profits of weight loss industry soar."

To bed. Maybe a little TV to help her relax. Tries a late-night talk show and is transfixed by the sight of audience members angrily attacking a man who's insulting his wife for being overweight. Then realizes there's nothing new here after all. Even when the intent is good, and sentiment seems to be on the side of a Fat Chick, it's still a given that she has commited a sin that must be repented and rectified. Switches to David Letterman: Fat Oprah Winfrey joke. Jay Leno: Fat Elizabeth Taylor joke. Some other clown: "Didja see where Roseanne . . ." Click.

And so to sleep. Perchance to dream that tomorrow won't be quite so full of hostility, humiliation, and hopelessness. Or that the miracle everyone's demanding of her will somehow happen overnight and she'll wake up slender.

Crazy or What?

This "day from hell" is an amalgam of experiences suffered by millions of large women, including me. All its horrid moments don't happen every day, thank heaven. But many do, and none more frequently than having your clock radio start the day off by letting you know you haven't a prayer of living prejudice-free any time soon, and at day's end falling asleep to TV's version of the same cruel "humor." And, in between, being clobbered by hostile stares and vulgar comments that head straight to your heart and stay there forever.

To be a target for this much grief, you probably have to weigh quite a lot, as I have for most of my life. But the essential point is that no one is propaganda-proof, whatever she weighs. The brainwashing is ubiquitous, and is perfectly characterized by Susan Douglas in *Where the Girls Are* as being bombarded with nonstop images of "smiling, air-brushed, anorexic, and compliant women whose message seems to be 'Shut up, get a face-lift, and stop eating.'"

And whenever we succumb to these outrageous slings and arrows by punitive dieting, "we turn our bodies into metaphors for all of our bad feelings—and we find confirmation for doing so everywhere we look," according to Jane R. Hirschmann and Carol H. Munter in their insightful book, *When Women Stop Hating Their Bodies: Freeing Yourself From Food and Weight Obsession.*

Has everyone gone crazy? Well, what else can we call it when

- we believe the body types of roughly 95 percent of the female population are abnormal and only the other 5 percent are acceptable;
- we act as if eating is perverted, antisocial behavior instead of something we all must do to stay alive;
- we blame the 95–98 percent failure rate of diets on dieters instead of applying basic cause-and-effect logic;
- we're oblivious to the epidemic of eating disorders and the plague of prejudice that's all around us;
- we're blind to the fundamental logic that if any of the diet schemes actually worked, all the others would go out of business;
- we're deaf to the messages of medical researchers about the counterproductivity of dieting and the implacability of genetic heredity;
- we ignore the elementary contradiction that, by trying to get thin, we're actually becoming fatter;
- like a nation of automatons, we epitomize the most basic definition of insanity—doing the same things over and over but expecting different results.

All this *sounds* like madness, but it's really just the logical result of three decades of brainwashing. Certainly, it's no accident that these

mass delusions flourish within a culture in which the mightiest industry of all manufactures anxiety, rather than steel or any other tangible.
But the hucksters who monopolize the mass media with their sheer
spending power have managed to create, escalate, and perpetuate
something far worse than mere anxiety about attractiveness or social
acceptability. During the post-Twiggy era, they have fostered epidemic
levels of not only the psycho-physiological illnesses of anorexia,
bulimia, and compulsive eating, but also the emotional maladies of
depression, paranoia, intolerance, fear, and body hatred—both self-
and other-directed.

No one under forty remembers it, but size diversity was just a fact
of life until the No Fat Chicks credo hooked us. Sure, some women
have always been considered more attractive than others, and those
others have always yearned to be deemed attractive. But until recently,
the less favored were never actually demonized or driven to psychological and physical self-destructiveness.

Today, Fat Chicks are the most blatantly reviled, ridiculed, and punished people in society. Fully twenty-five years after the women's liberation movement galvanized us into achieving our potential in so
many other ways, the most treasured goal of the majority of women—
according to numerous surveys—is not personal fulfillment, family
love, professional success, or wealth, but simply becoming as tiny as
the bogus beauty icons paraded past us every waking moment.

Incredible as it seems, no authorities are monitoring the emotional toll
on the millions of women whose response to the societal demand for
thinness is extremely dangerous behavior. The resulting dearth of data
forces me to extrapolate from general psychological research on
women—which, in itself, is extremely sobering. The fact is, "in every
culture that has this ideal of thinness, depression is twice as common
for women as for men, and there are more incidences of eating disorders," according to psychologist Martin E. P. Seligman, author of *What
You Can Change and What You Can't.*

American women, too, suffer from major depression and manic-
depressive disorder at twice the rate of men (25 percent, as compared
with 12 percent) and receive an estimated 83 percent of all antidepressants prescribed by psychiatrists, and an incredible 90 percent

of tranquilizers and other psychotropic medications prescribed by
other types of doctors, according to a shocking book, *Outrageous Practices: The Alarming Truth About How Medicine Mistreats Women*, by
Leslie Laurence and Beth Weinhouse.

What I know personally about being a Fat Chick, together with
everything I learned in the course of researching this book, convinced
me beyond doubt that a huge number of large women are among
these millions of depressed, psychologically maltreated patients. In
fact—given that we are often humiliated on a daily basis from childhood onward, and then deprived of fulfilling lives—the psychological
cost is, arguably, even worse: We have a sky-high rate of severe depression, an abysmally low level of self-esteem, and a profound sense of
disempowerment and hopelessness.

And Fat Chicks also pay a concomitant physical price, as evidenced
by a recent study at the University of California at Irvine, which
determined that chronic emotional distress is an even worse health
risk than smoking, and actually doubles a person's chances of incurring serious disease.

Why such a heavy toll? "Because you can't measure up to [the] cultural ideal, you feel unworthy. You just want to go away and hide,"
explains Judith Jordan, Ph.D., director of the Women's Treatment
Network at McLean Hospital in Belmont, Massachusetts. "But you
can't—when you're overweight, it's broadcast to the world. And you
get caught in [a] spiral of social withdrawal, becoming more isolated
and ashamed."

What's the best way of communicating how helpless all this makes
an overweight woman feel? Maybe by borrowing a dramatic technique
used in a crisis shelter near my home. To give volunteers and visitors
some insight into the perplexing question of why women stay in abusive relationships, staffers haul out a huge stack of heavy wool blankets. Someone steps forward and is gradually covered by blanket after
blanket after blanket, until she can no longer see or hear anything outside her dark cocoon, until she can hardly breathe, and until the
weight is so heavy she cannot move, let alone find an escape route.

The blankets represent the layers of fear and psychological undermining that insidiously trap abused women. In our fat-phobic society,
large women are just as entangled inside layers of prejudice and emo-

tional distress. But the psychological fall-out from living in a society that hates you and teaches you to hate yourself garners very little serious, or even respectful, professional attention. Why? Because the Fat Chick's problems are thought to be voluntarily incurred, personally remediable, and essentially trivial.

Eloquent testimony about the toll all this takes turned up in many of the responses to my Internet queries and *USA Today* ad:

GAIL: They taught me to see myself as grotesque. That's not accurate but it's apparently what they see, and that's all that counts in this world.

TESS: What's toughest for me is realizing that this whole thing has kept me from appreciating my own good qualities: I don't smoke, drink, carouse, gamble, overspend, or emotionally abuse anybody. I'm healthy, strong, honest, brave, idealistic, and I have tons of willpower. Yet others' perception of me is the opposite, so I keep thinking: How can I be right and the rest of the world be wrong?

CARRIE: I read about a Scottish study of how depressed people get when they don't win the lottery. And I thought: that's one of the reasons it's so devastating to keep on trying to lose weight. Every time you step on a scale and see that you haven't lost anything, you feel more hopeless than the time before.

Identity Crisis

"I am ... invisible ... simply because people refuse to see me. ... When they approach me, they see only my surroundings, themselves, or figments of their imagination—indeed, everything and anything except me."

So wrote renowned novelist Ralph Ellison about being black fifty years ago. But his eloquent description applies equally well to Fat Chicks. When you're noticeably overweight, you suffer the double whammy of disappearing, as far as your real identity is concerned, yet remaining all too visible as an object of disgust. It's a very disorienting clash of feelings—like being naked in public and feeling humiliated because of it. Yet, at the same time, you feel as though what people are seeing isn't the real you. It's a disguise you never chose, yet it's attracting more punishment than is heaped upon anyone else in our society.

> JUDY: They refuse to recognize who you really are. It's like you're invisible even though everybody's staring at you in disgust. And even if they do finally see you, they insist that you be what they insist on seeing. And they can get very angry if you won't play along.
>
> DENITRA: There are only a few acceptable roles for us: buffoon, whipping girl, object lesson. And about all people will tolerate from us is if we're jolly or obsequious.
>
> DEIRDRE: It's gotten to where I feel so disconnected from this body everybody hates that I've stopped wishing to be thin. Now I want to be invisible, just pure spirit.

Many Fat Chicks respond to the condemnation they endure in this "looks above all" world by attempting to do psychological penance. They mentally accept their designation as cultural criminals and sentence themselves accordingly to virtual solitary confinement. This consists of not just isolation from others, but also putting their lives "on hold" in what Geneen Roth has dubbed the "When I'm Thin Fantasy." "We've told ourselves that the reason we're not loved properly is our fault for not being thin," she writes in *When Food Is Love*. "Blaming ourselves gives us a feeling of some control [and] the illusion that when we're finally thin, we will be loved properly." Until that magical day arrives, many women—both the truly overweight and those who falsely believe they are too heavy—unconsciously fend off every opportunity that might lead to acquiring husbands, children, and normal social lives.

Why is their need for control so intense? Because to be obese is to feel out of control, to know that you are considered unstable by others, and to be defied by your own body, which refuses to obey, no matter how hard you drive it. Also, of course, our sexist, market-driven culture guarantees that all women's bodies are considered common commodities.

> PEGGY: How can women have the slightest hope of recovering from the disease of body hate when we live in a culture that's completely toxic?

FRAN: It offends me that women are supposed to be so small—not just skinny, but really teensy. I always remember what Roseanne says: that women should get bigger, not smaller, until we take up so much space that we'll have to be taken seriously.

There is no escape from the scrutiny, even if you're talented, famous, and successful. Just ask actresses Sharon Gless and Tyne Daly, whose mutual weight gain, though modest, was widely remarked when they reprised their *Cagney & Lacey* series as TV specials. Or the lead singers of Heart and Fleetwood Mac, whose respective chubbiness was the subject of far more comments than their voices when their groups reunited. Or country singer Wynonna Judd, whose size is often a target for snide or pitying remarks in popular magazines, and who was humiliated in front of millions of people recently when *Tonight* show host Jay Leno inexplicably tried to pick her up after she sang a song—and both of them tumbled to the floor.

Or check with the only female national leader on this continent to date, former Canadian prime minister Kim Campbell. Vulgar comments about what was actually a very moderate weight gain were made by colleagues and by the media throughout her short-lived administration.

Linda Ronstadt's plumpness as she approaches age fifty is mentioned by practically every disc jockey who introduces her records. Even when *Mirabella* magazine published an otherwise flattering article about her recently, writer Karen Schoemer and her editors chose to include a put-down that revealed their own class bias: "Ronstadt has put on a good deal of weight, and in workout clothes she more closely resembles a woman in front of you in the supermarket checkout line than the most successful female pop star of the seventies."

CONNIE: What kind of a sick world is it where the only "legitimate" accomplishment for a woman is denying her most basic needs and starving herself so she'll get smaller and smaller?

Other plus-size women—especially those whose self-esteem is comparatively intact—grapple with different psychological obstacles. Some long to be slender, but bitterly resent the pressure to conform. So their answer to those who tell women to squash themselves into ever tinier packages is a defiant no. But this means that, in their own minds, they're damned if they do lose weight and damned if they don't.

Then there are the deal makers, whose state of mind is eloquently expressed by Pam Houston in *Minding the Body—Women Writers on Body and Soul*: "For a good part of my life, I would have quite literally given anything to be thin . . . a finger, three toes, the sight in one eye. Now I find it only mildly surprising that for the majority of my lifetime I would have traded being ugly, deformed, and thin for being pretty, whole, and fat."

Similarly, a University of Florida study of women who'd lost weight after intestinal-bypass surgery reported that virtually all said they'd rather be blind, deaf, or have a leg amputated than ever be fat again. If this seems incongruous, remember that, today, the highest form of compliment is congratulating a woman for squashing herself to a smaller size.

But Why's Everybody Else So Mad?

The other side of the coin, in terms of what the billion-dollar brainwash has wrought, is the intense anger so many people feel toward Fat Chicks. Certainly, other minorities face deplorable prejudice. But when you're overweight, the hostility feels more personally directed. After all, nobody is told flat out to switch religions, or to change the color of her skin or the contour of her facial features. The disabled aren't ordered to shape up, and those with diseases aren't told to simply snap out of it. Society has finally evolved to the point where alcoholics, drug addicts, and the mentally ill are generally treated with compassion instead of contempt. But the overweight are still regarded as *deserving* of abuse and exclusion.

Why? Because our society has been deliberately conditioned to be repelled by the very sight of a fat woman. This knee-jerk reaction is constantly reinforced in the media—both information and entertainment—by means of the hundreds of images that surround us during an average day. Yet a stroll through any traditional art gallery will confirm that this is a conditioned, rather than a primary, response, and that it is of very recent vintage.

Oddly enough, however, appearance per se isn't the most significant element of the taboo against obesity, according to many psychological authorities. Rather, the hostility has more to do with the presumed breaking of rules that others feel compelled to obey. Given that the majority of women are not naturally thin, especially as they age, achieving this body image takes prodigious effort and self-denial. Yet only rarely do we hear *unnaturally* slender women characterize this as the extreme sacrifice it is. And even when they do hint at it, they blame themselves instead of the ruthless pressure to accomplish the impossible. In fact, it's often as if a societal ventriloquist is at work when they alternately apologize for eating and concoct absurd rationalizations for consuming even innocuous amounts.

What's the reaction when someone who has gone to punitive lengths to be slim sees someone who evidently has not? Anger, because the Fat Chick appears to be enjoying the pleasures her slender sisters are denying themselves. Even worse is the implicit assumption that she's not only not playing the game, but actually repudiating the rules and ridiculing those who abide by them. So, as feminist scholar Susan Bordo phrases it in *Unbearable Weight: Feminism, Western Culture and the Body*: "If the rest of us are struggling to be acceptable and 'normal,' we cannot allow [the obese] to get away with it; they must be put in their place . . . humiliated and defeated."

KALLI: The truth is that very, very few people have enough will-power to starve themselves for years and years, let alone do all the other stuff I do to lose weight. Yet I'm treated as if I'm a lazy slug with no self-control at all.

PAULA: I keep trying to think of a way to buttonhole these people who obviously hate how I look, and say, "You're wrong. This is not the body I gorged my way up to, it's the one I got by a lifetime of starving to please you."

The resentment is exacerbated when an overweight woman seems to be contented with her size, or when her demeanor indicates that she expects to be treated respectfully.

KATH: Nobody expects blacks to shuffle any more. But if [fat women] just have a normal amount of self-confidence or dignity, people are outraged. How dare we expect to be treated like human beings?

Another basis for anger-inducing antifat prejudice is what I call the Dorian Gray Syndrome, borrowing from Oscar Wilde's famous tale about a man who remained handsome while the physical evidence of his depravity appeared on an increasingly hideous portrait. I believe this scenario is reenacted whenever slim people project onto Fat Chicks the qualities they've been brainwashed into believing are the ugliest, but fear they themselves embody. What qualities? Gluttony, sloth, selfishness, asexuality, lack of control, lack of self-respect, unfemininity. The inference is that "anyone who allows herself to be or become fat is exhibiting in a public way weaknesses or flaws in her basic nature," as Jane Rachel Kaplan explains in *A Woman's Conflict: The Special Relationship Between Women and Food*, adding that "persons who exhibit such imperfection are not living up to the standards of decency followed by all other members of the society, and therefore do not deserve to share equally in the rewards offered by the system."

This process of "trial by appearance" is often subconscious. But many (naturally and unnaturally) slender women embrace the No Fat Chicks rule itself quite consciously—which brings to mind what crusader Elizabeth Cady Stanton said of those who opposed female suffrage in the late nineteenth century: "It is too bad that these women are begging to be left in their chains."

> CINDY: We've got to realize that all this insistence on women having perfect bodies is as insulting and regressive as if we suddenly had to start coming up with dowries of so many cows or goats.

Even Losers Can't Win

Ironically, a Fat Chick can incur anger from others even when she does manage to "go with the flow" by losing weight. A troubled woman named Connie, for example, told the authors of *When Women Stop Hating Their Bodies* that, after losing quite a lot, she realized "that not only have I been eating differently, I've been acting differently as well. . . . [And] I suspect that [the] real problem has more to do with the fact that I'm not as compliant as I once was . . ."

It wasn't Connie's new figure but her newfound self-respect that landed her in hot water at home. As strange as it seems, Fat Chicks' significant others—even those who insist upon slimness—often try to sabotage the dieting process as soon as results reach a significant level. This may take the form of insisting a dieter looks better when she's heavier; warning her that she's endangering her health; criticizing her for not providing adequate meals for other members of the household; or inundating her environment with fattening food. One of the reasons I found it necessary to move away from home while doing my magazine diet series was that the (previously abstemious) man I lived with suddenly began hauling home donuts and other "treats."

Why the contradictory signals? Because relational change is often frightening. So the perception (which may be conscious or subconscious) is that the balance of power in relationships will be upset if the woman no longer considers herself inferior. And the status quo is equally threatened if her popularity outside the home increases.

So even when a Fat Chick succeeds in losing a substantial amount of weight, her problems are far from over. Among the challenges she'll likely face are coping with domestic hostility; combating the physical fail-safe mechanism described in Chapter 3; and fighting to overcome the residual psychological fear and bitterness instilled while she was a target for prejudice.

Another problem may be discomfort because of the loss of the "invisible cloak" provided by fatness which, even while drawing disapproval, may protect a heavy woman from unwanted attention. Thomas F. Cash, author of *What Do You See When You Look in the Mirror*, writes about women who were severely disturbed by being hooted at by construction workers and other strangers after they'd lost weight.

There's also what's termed the scapegoat effect, which refers to the tendency to attribute all one's difficulties—personal, social, and career—to being overweight. When the pounds disappear, so does the scapegoat, often leaving confusion in its wake.

Still another demon a newly slim woman may have to wrestle is called body-image distortion. The most extreme form of this inability to really see the new body that's reflected in the mirror affects anorexics, who somehow perceive phantom flab where there's actually nothing except skin and bones. But other formerly fat women also have a tough time believing their eyes and therefore appreciating that they've reached their cherished goal.

This kind of bewilderment happened to me in a clothing store when I was searching for something to wear for a TV appearance following my magazine diet series. Holding a dress three sizes smaller than anything I'd worn since my teens, I panicked when I saw a sales clerk approach. Years of being insulted or ignored by her ilk made me jump to the conclusion that she was going to snatch the dress out of my hands and revile me for thinking it would fit. Instead, she smiled graciously and suggested I needed an even smaller size. She was right, yet somehow I still couldn't see my body realistically.

The Worst Punishment

Ironically, cruelty from an increasingly intolerant world isn't the worst part of being overweight. Even more painful is the internalization of the No Fat Chicks edict that leads obese women to feel guilty, ashamed, and worthless every day of their lives—an experience which feels, to quote an e-mail note from a woman named Molly, "like swimming upstream in a river of burning molasses."

Even Oprah Winfrey, the most successful and admired woman on television, felt psychologically crushed when the weight she lost so publicly during her liquid-protein fast crept back. "I'm 180 pounds," she wrote in 1990 in one of many such journal entries. "Now I wake every morning hating myself." When she won an Emmy award, Winfrey says she felt so ashamed of being "the fattest woman in the room . . . waddl[ing] my way up to the stage with the nation watching my huge behind" that she didn't want to accept it.

But even those whose innate good sense lets them reject most of the ghastly qualities projected onto overweight women are still vulnerable to the negativity of the people in their lives who *do* think this way and treat them accordingly—especially in all the ways described in the foregoing "day from hell." Care to guess whether that helps? Never mind. Psychologist and eating-disorders specialist Susan Wooley has come up with the heartbreakingly definitive answer: "If shame could cure obesity, there wouldn't be a fat person in the world."

To Eat or Not to Eat

The mere presence of food can sometimes spell psychological torture for Fat Chicks and for those who fear being thus defined. To eat or not to eat is the question that can buzz incessantly in the brain. Why? Because food can simultaneously represent the temptation of a taboo, as well as both the catalyst for your persecution, and the source of consolation from that persecution. So the murky emotional ratio of hating, loving, and needing food means that simply knowing it's nearby can induce subliminal panic similar to that we face before a crucial exam. In conflicted moments like this, I have often felt as if I were walking a tightrope and it was a given that I'd eventually fall. The suspense of whether this would happen sooner rather than later could be unbearable.

But what about the millions of North American women whose response to societal pressures is to develop clinical eating disorders, including anorexia (refusal to eat), bulimia (bingeing followed by purging), and compulsive eating? Paradoxically, large women whose compulsive eating has become out of control actually represent the flip side of an anorexic's rejection of food. Both are eating-disorder victims who believe this is the only arena in their lives they can control. But the skinny woman says no to food, while the fat one is often saying yes, not out of gluttony, but out of a need to mentally counterbalance all the other no's she hears from society because of her size.

Others who are battling their weight often form a powerful dependence on foods that represent comfort. Why? One illuminating answer comes, not from an unhappy housewife in the hinterlands, but from a beautiful, celebrated actress, Elizabeth Taylor, whose weight nearly doubled during her unhappy marriage to a politician. "The large amounts of food I ate were a substitute for everything I felt I was lacking in my life. But what was really starving was my self-esteem."

As for anorexia, there are many theories about the cause, including the one that seems most obvious to me: simply "overconforming" to society's demand for thin women. As historian Joan Jacobs Brumberg writes in *Fasting Girls: The Emergence of Anorexia Nervosa as a Modern Disease* (the preeminent book in this field): "Given our longstanding and extravagant collective worship at the shrine of slimness, it is no wonder that so many contemporary young women make dieting an article of faith and that anorexia nervosa has become the characteristic psychopathology of the female adolescent of our day."

And the tragic ultimate stage for an anorexic, as psychotherapist Kim Chernin writes in *The Obsession: Reflections on the Tyranny of Slenderness*, is "a feeling of profound humiliation that the body exists at all."

About bulimia, which authorities say is even less curable than anorexia, there seems to be a virtual consensus that the behavior is a psychological "adjustment" to the pressures of fat-phobia. Chernin focuses on bulimics, to powerful effect, in another of her excellent books. In *The Hungry Self: Women, Eating and Identity*, she quotes a study of normally functioning college women who "[experience] their hunger as exaggerated and obscene," and describes the eating obsessions of many of her patients. The most compelling case study is that of a patient Chernin calls Anita, who told her that, because of the all-consuming pressure to be thin, "[we women] are vomiting our guts out to let [society] know we just can't stomach it." The day after singer Karen Carpenter died of anorexia, the patient told Chernin: "Now they'll *have* to take it seriously."

Sorry to say it, but Anita was wrong. A decade after *The Hungry Self* was published, the number of American women and girls with eating disorders has soared above 11 million and is still rising. Many of these women—especially those of college age—readily admit that staying slim is their motive for starving themselves or vomiting much of what they eat, and that they frequently accompany this behavior with laxative and diuretic abuse and compulsive overexercising—not to mention swelling the ranks of the fastest-growing category of smokers in the country.

"Restrained eating" is considered by some authorities to be a fourth kind of eating disorder. But, as asserted by University of Toronto researchers Janet Polivy and C. Peter Herman, who coined the term, the practice of permanently limiting your food intake to less than you desire is now so commonplace that many experts (not to mention the general public) don't think of it as a disorder at all. "The meaning of a phrase such as normal eating," the duo wrote in a 1987 article in the *Journal of Consulting and Clinical Psychology*, "is no longer obvious [because] 'normal' eating for North American women is now characterized by dieting."

And what's the effect of obsessive restrained eating—always saying no to yourself and feeling permanently deprived? I can think of no better answer than to quote another of Oscar Wilde's brilliant observations. We've all heard the first line many times, but the second part—which is so significant in this context—is rarely repeated: "The only way to get rid of temptation is to yield to it. Resist it, and your soul grows sick with longing for the things it has forbidden to itself."

The Big Question

No discussion of the psychological toll exacted by the billion-dollar brainwash would be complete without addressing the basic question that seems to mystify so many "normal-weight" people and prompt so much prejudice: Why do Fat Chicks choose to be miserable misfits by staying so much bigger than they "should" be? Answer: They don't. In fact, the ultimate defeat for Fat Chicks is that incessant dieting actually keeps them fat (a process described in Chapter 3).

The Big Lie—that obesity must be voluntary because anyone who tries hard enough can be permanently thin—is one of the most cunning ploys adopted by the antifat profiteers. But the rock-bottom truth is that the media version of slenderness is simply not a possibility for many body types. It is a "myth that we can force our bodies into the shape we think they ought to be," says Dr. Jane Blouin, a psychologist at Ottawa Civic Hospital's eating-disorder clinic. "It doesn't work that way any more than you can force your foot into the size of shoe you want."

Now think about it. What could possibly be more psychologically devastating than to keep doing what everyone in the world is demanding, over and over again, year after desperate year, only to have the supposed solution turn out to be an inescapable trap?

As we've seen, then, the current epidemic of obesity, eating disorders, and depression is chiefly the result of deliberate disinformation, carefully instilled fat-phobia, and the inescapable imperative for incessant dieting. Yet, just as obviously, there *are* other complicated causes.

Physically, excess weight is often the result of such factors as genetic heredity, food intolerances, and insulin imbalance. In many other cases, the paramount causation is emotional, with obesity and eating disorders being not so much the problem as the sad solution. Such cases include survivors of sexual abuse—possibly as many as 50–60 percent of the total, according to a study cited by Dr. Kathryn J. Zerbe in *The Body Betrayed: Women, Eating Disorders and Treatment*. Not only do such women consider eating the safest source of comfort, they also know that, in our current culture, nothing advertises a woman's sexual unavailability, or repels potential partners, more effectively than a protective layer of fat.

> SANDRA: I've come to think of my body as my disguise. It's my cave and my bomb shelter. And it's my walking rebuke to those who inflict Barbie doll demands on all women.

An inability to handle anger appropriately can also result in overeating, so that women try to "stuff" their rage down deep. Why are they so angry? According to many experts, it's frequently because of physical, sexual, and emotional abuse or neglect, especially in childhood. The logical outcome of feeling betrayed and abandoned, as author and former compulsive eater Geneen Roth puts it in *When Food Is Love*, is the fear "that if I didn't eat, I was giving up an opportunity, maybe my last, to fill the part of me that was forever hungry, forever desperate for relief. I could never honestly say that I had enough because although my body was full, I was empty."

Substituting food for emotional nurturance that's otherwise unavailable is also aptly described by an overweight woman in Marcia Millman's *Such a Pretty Face: Being Fat in America*: "I'm trying to be a good neighbor and a good daughter and a good parent and a good wife and a good teacher and a good scholar and a good friend and the one thing that will take care of me is food."

Psychiatrist Theodore Isaac Rubin provides yet another description of the motivation for overeating comfort foods in *Alive and Fat and Thinning in America*: "In an attempt to ward off depression, fat people will eat . . . to counter sadness with pleasure . . . to feel love and warmth symbolized by foods and memories of maternal care expressed through feeding. . . . Thus, eating binges are often . . . defenses against depression."

Makes sense, right? But let's get real here. How many people *don't* equate food with nurturance and use it to assuage emotional turmoil?

We're all programmed that way, not only by cultural conditioning, but by the fact that eating boosts the level of the neurotransmitter serotonin in the brain, producing a feeling of well-being. Yet those whose extra pounds make them walking advertisements for this elementary human dynamic are treated as if their behavior is destructive, aberrant, irresponsible, and unforgivable.

And the kicker is that, even though eating, as Zerbe points out in *The Body Betrayed*, "functions as a form of self-medication against painful feelings ... [in people who] suffer mightily in many areas of their lives," bigotry has deprived so many fat people of other rewarding life experiences, including having companions or children. Yet the one source of consolation that's available on every corner—food—is what they alone are expected to do without.

> IRENE: What I hate most are all those makeover articles in the magazines. It's like we're surrounded by all this stuff telling us how to be somebody else. And, of course, on all the other pages, it's diets, diets, diets on one side of the page and humongous pictures of food on the other side. It's crazy, but nobody even notices the contradiction.

Yeah, but . . .

Okay, fine, but why do the remainder of Fat Chicks eat? To stay alive. That sounds ridiculously obvious, but think about it. Somewhere along the way, we seem to have forgotten that—however much she may regret, or be despised for, her appearance—the heavy woman cannot quit "cold turkey." She *must* eat, 365 days a year. Just like everyone else. Yet unlike others, her ability to know when she is truly hungry or truly full may have been destroyed by years of heeding, not her body's signals, but external dictates, especially the arbitrary do's and don'ts of typical diet regimens.

Beyond that, of course, is the inescapable social obligation and familial ritual of eating. When do we ever get together for a cup of nothing? Or sit around a nice empty table celebrating a holiday? As a prominent food anthropologist puts it, "In all societies, both simple and complex, eating is the primary way of initiating and maintaining human relationships."

Mustn't we agree, then, that the Fat Chick's basic motivations for consuming food match those of every other human being since the beginning of time? Ah, but not everybody eats enough to get fat, right? Actually, a growing percentage of us do, especially since regular sit-down meals have been all but supplanted by frequent "grazing" on fast and fatty foods. And this has been exacerbated by the dramatic decrease in physical activity in modern times, to the point where a third of all Americans now weigh at least 20 percent more than is currently approved.

So Fat Chicks aren't abnormal after all. They're simply the most visible products of our culture and our cultural conditioning. Left unchecked, the marketers who manipulate these forces will continue manufacturing all the consumers they need for their worthless wares.

Bottom Line

The foregoing illustrates what a sea of psychological trouble Fat Chicks are forced to swim in every day. And, just to make it worse, when they turn to medical or psychological practitioners for help with the sharks that besiege them, all they usually get are insults, lectures, and diet sheets.

Even enormously famous and successful women are unable to escape the No Fat Chicks imperative. Those whose resultant eating disorders have become public knowledge include Princess Diana; *Beauty Myth* author Naomi Wolf; dancers Paula Abdul and Gelsey Kirkland; the late singer Karen Carpenter; comedian Joan Rivers; and actresses Jane Fonda, Sally Field, Lynn Redgrave, Janine Turner, the late Gilda Radner, Tracey Gold, who was fired from the *Growing Pains* TV series because of uncontrollable anorexia, and *Married With Children* star Christina Applegate, who told *People* magazine that she eats only when she's "doubled over and passing out."

In the introduction to this book, I described the abrupt psychological shock of losing my "golden girl" status when I became fat in pre-pubescence. Until then, it seemed as if everyone loved me—and, afterward, that no one did, or ever would. As I continued writing, I forced myself to review the many cruel words and gestures that have stayed with me for a lifetime. Soon even bitter memories I'd managed to repress for decades floated back into my consciousness. Example: At age twelve, I was so ashamed of my tubby tummy that I secretly kept a tight, rubbery girdle on under my pajamas at my first slumber party. I was so uncomfortable and afraid that the other girls would find me out that I couldn't sleep all night and crept away at dawn.

Another unwelcome recollection cost me a few nights' sleep when I reflected on, not just my childhood pain, but the consequence of being among the high percentage of fat teenage girls who are too demoralized to pursue higher education. Why? Because of humiliations that begin in grade school and never stop. Example: Being forced to compete in grotesque sports competitions, called "field days." I was inevitably among the least capable pupils attempting compulsory races, jumps, and other feats that were far too difficult for those of us who were overweight, puny, or congenitally uncoordinated. The ordeal was intensified by always being scheduled last, which meant that, with our families and the entire student body watching, we were an annual spectacle in our small town. And whichever of us came in last—often me—was taunted by the other kids throughout the following year as the "worst of the worst."

I was forcibly reminded of how hurtful it is to be such an overweight child while watching a recent television special called *Growing Up Fat*. A dozen or so teenagers who had spent many summers trying to lose weight at "fat camps" were filmed as they watched a videotape showing a class of five-year-olds boisterously exhibiting the antifat prejudice that had already been instilled in them. The teenagers' expressions as they listened to the younger kids shouting that stupidity, ugliness, and even mutilation are preferable to obesity were utterly heartbreaking.

The fact is, the billion-dollar brainwash has created communicable forms of madness to which precious few are now immune. So unless it can be stopped, life will continue to be emotionally anguished and needlessly restricted for any of these youngsters who actually grow up to be Fat Chicks or who merely live in fear of doing so.

And that's the whole idea—because every time they respond by trying to reduce, somewhere a cash register will ca-ching up another chunk of the unconscionable profits that derive from mass delusion.

5

Doctor Feel-Bads

....

In *Sleeper*, Woody Allen's quirky comedy about a man who's thawed out after two hundred years of cryogenic sleep, a couple of chain-smoking physicians chat about how amazingly misguided their professional ancestors were. In the twentieth century, says one, doctors actually thought steak, ice cream, and smoking were *bad* for people. The second quack shakes her head in amazement and takes another puff.

I wish I had something equally droll to say about the medical community's philosophical seesawing on the topic of obesity. But there's nothing amusing about the fact that those whose sworn duty is to protect our health have mostly snoozed, squabbled, or profiteered during the past three decades, allowing the billion-dollar brainwash to flourish unimpeded.

Actually, I *do* know a sick joke. Only thing is, it's true. Ready? Some doctors are starting to make house calls again, and even office calls. But they're *not* trekking all over creation to tend to sick people; they're hustling out to scribble prescriptions for the wildly popular new diet "wonder drugs."

Those *most* culpable in the creation of prejudice-for-profit, as we've seen in previous chapters, are the actual peddlers of weight loss products, and the advertisers and media vehicles that help them vilify Fat Chicks and traumatize all other females. But there's plenty of blame left over for those who either stand silently by while all this happens, or enthusiastically hop aboard the money wagon themselves.

The worst of the "unindicted coconspirators" who aid, abet, or passively countenance the antifat industry are in the medical profession, especially the country's 17,500 "bariatric" physicians,* and the 3,300 hospitals that specialize in weight loss. Am I exaggerating about their complicity? You tell me, after asking why physicians haven't yet seen through the No Fat Chicks charade and called a halt—especially after several major authorities officially declared that obesity is not a moral failing, but a disease.

The answer *has* to be that "fat people are waddling reminders of the failure of medicine to come to a safe, workable program for long-term weight reduction, just as poor people and homeless people are stark reminders of the failure of the economic system." The charge is made in *Never Satisfied: A Cultural History of Diets, Fantasies and Fat* by author Hillel Schwartz, who adds the scathing comment that, "like politicians, physicians blame the victims."

For the record, let me repeat that excess weight *can* be a health hazard for many individuals, especially those who are extremely heavy, and *may* lead to heart disease, diabetes, and some cancers. Nothing I have written is meant to contradict this. But the topic addressed here is *not* the legitimate physical consequences of obesity; it's the false claims and psychological coercion used by profiteers to dupe virtually the entire population of the United States.

Nevertheless, in terms of the "big picture," the majority of Americans are now overweight, and national obesity-related health-care costs are estimated at a whopping $100 billion, making this the second-worst national risk category (after smoking). I have no way of knowing how this figure was arrived at, or how accurate it is. But there's no question that it's a stinging indictment of fat people, right? Not necessarily. Before blindly accepting this assumption, we must consider three relevant factors.

*The Americal Medical Association does not recognize "bariatrics" as a genuine specialty, and therefore its practitioners have no obligation to qualify for certification.

One: That the lion's share of the blame for creating this situation belongs, as we saw in previous chapters, far less to individual self-indulgence than to the propaganda machine that incessantly baits an array of traps to ensure that millions of people get fat and stay that way.

Two: Simple knee-jerk reasoning, as Marcia Millman expresses it in *Such a Pretty Face: Being Fat in America,* fails to take into account the fact that "fat people are blamed for problems and expenses [that are actually] created by the structure of our medical care system and its profit orientation. Blame for the failure of the health system is shifted to individuals who are actually more its victims than its perpetrators."

Three: The source for that sky-high estimate of weight-related health-care costs is former surgeon general C. Everett Koop. While I have no evidence suggesting that he is anything but sincere in his desire for a healthier populace, the fact is that the organization Dr. Koop now fronts—called Shape Up America—is largely funded by Weight Watchers, which, in turn, is owned by the H. J. Heinz food conglomerate. And it was this giant company that recently chose Koop as the recipient of the $250,000 Heinz Award for his work on behalf of enhancing public health.*

In addition, the late 1994 news conference during which Koop announced the formation of Shape Up America and denounced the gluttony and laziness which he cited as the causes of rampant obesity, was called mere days after widespread headlines about the discovery of the "ob gene." Again, as a layperson, I have no way of evaluating the data concerning this purported breakthrough. But I certainly *can* infer, from excitement within the scientific community, that the identification of a gene that causes excess weight levels may eventually lead to the elimination of fatness altogether. By logical extension, this will one day mean the loss of the profiteers' $50 billion annual fortune.

To be completely explicit here, what I'm saying is that we've got to ask ourselves a cogent question: If *we* owned the largest weight loss organization in the world—Weight Watchers—and our membership had been dropping by 15 to 25 percent annually since 1989, wouldn't

---

Rump Parliament, a feisty size-acceptance publication described in Chapter 10, made its opinion crystal clear by publishing a cartoon depicting Koop as a hand puppet operated by the weight loss industry.

we have a vital stake in convincing everyone that obesity is their worst enemy?

Yet, even more to the point, the startling truth the antifat profiteers don't want us to know—and few physicians ever admit—is that "fat" and "fit" are *not* mutually exclusive terms. Extra weight is actually beneficial in various medical circumstances. And ample evidence supporting this heretical point of view is now turning up in study after study, as we will see in a moment.

But even if being overweight *were* unequivocally unhealthy—to both individuals and the economy—it's no contradiction to say that doctors should have done something to mitigate the forced march in the wrong direction dictated by the billion-dollar brainwash. The medical profession has been on the front lines of the phenomenon. Doctors and other professionals have seen their patients' obsession and misery at first hand, and they possess the professional expertise to judge what is happening.

Or, rather, what *isn't* happening.

Instead of becoming permanently thinner by dieting, millions of women are steadily growing fatter, and suffering physically and emotionally along the way. Other patients stay slim only because they avoid nutritious food such as milk, develop anorexia or bulimia, or deliberately court disaster by smoking to curb their appetites,* or popping excessive amounts of diet drugs, amphetamines, diuretics, laxatives, and even antidepressants such as Prozac. And countless other women have succumbed to hopelessness, as well as hostility from their doctors, by ceasing to seek medical treatment at all.

Why haven't doctors noticed all this? Or interpreted it correctly? Or evidently even cared? There are only a few possible reasons and, I'm sorry to say, they all have ugly names.

Let's start with *prejudice*. The worst example of this I can cite is so over the top you may have trouble believing it. I know I did, even when it happened to me while I was appearing on a national TV talk show after the Canadian release of *No Fat Chicks*. One of my fellow panelists was Dr. Kenneth Walker, a Toronto G.P. who writes a nation-

---

*To the extent that lung cancer now exceeds breast cancer as a leading cause of death among women.

ally syndicated newspaper column under the pseudonym "Gifford-
Jones." Sitting right beside me, and speaking live to an audience of
millions, Walker repeated, without humor or irony, a notion he'd
already written in his column: that, for their own good, and for the
good of the national health budget, overweight people should be
locked up in prison camps.

Mercifully, that shocking degree of bigotry is rare. But if you ask
any Fat Chick about the treatment she gets from doctors, you'll likely
get an earful about the antipathy, mistrust, indifference, and downright
contempt with which she is often treated. And this is in addition to the
dismal situation that all female patients find themselves in, according
to the 1993 Commonwealth Fund study, which found that one out of
every four women is "talked down to" by doctors, while one out of five
is told that her problems are "all in her head." Another study, at the
University of Rochester, concluded that the average length of time
patients (of both sexes) are allowed to speak before being interrupted
by their physicians is a scant eighteen seconds.

But it's even worse for Fat Chicks. Some physicians refuse to treat
them at all until they lose weight. Others grow angry when patients fail
to achieve or sustain weight loss. Some don't bother with such elementary tasks as using large-size blood pressure cuffs to obtain accurate readings on fat arms. And no matter what ailment a large woman
has, medical personnel often either imply that it's related to her obesity, or ignore her actual complaints and address themselves solely to
her weight. This is roughly akin to taking your car into the shop
because of a faulty carburetor but being told there's no use even discussing your problem until you get a new paint job.

I can personally attest to most of these discriminatory practices.
When I consulted a doctor about my broken ankle a few years ago, for
example, he told me to walk the length of a corridor. I assumed he was
assessing the impairment of my gait, but when I turned around, I saw
that he was blatantly looking me up and down. "Have you ever thought
about getting your stomach stapled?" he asked. Then he sat me down,
drew a picture of a stomach showing where the staples are placed, and
handed me the name and phone number of a surgeon. When he
finally got around to discussing my ankle, the doctor implied that the
accident that caused it must have been caused by my excess weight—

a ludicrous notion, as he'd have realized if he'd bothered to listen to my explanation.

Gynecologists are among the worst offenders of all, according to a recent report to the Medical and Health Research Association. Examples included a traumatized woman who was brought to a hospital by police after being raped, and then was harangued about her weight by the doctor examining her for legal evidence; and another patient who, while seeking a birth control prescription, was asked who could possibly be interested in having sex with her, except maybe whale-hunting Captain Ahab. I will never forget my own humiliation when a gynecologist roughly prodded my stomach and complained about having to examine me "through all this upholstery."

What can possibly account for such a massive dereliction of duty on the part of people who sincerely devote themselves to the caring profession? It's the "Lose 50 Pounds and Call Me in the Morning" syndrome, says biomedical researcher Dr. Paul Ernsberger, author of "Rethinking Obesity: An Alternative View of Its Health Implications," a special issue of the *Journal of Obesity and Weight Regulation*. In it, he cites studies revealing that "one third of family practice doctors admit to feelings of discomfort, distaste or hostility when treating obese patients." Ernsberger's contention is amplified by the results of a national survey published in the *Journal of Family Practitioners* which indicated that a majority of the respondent doctors consider obese patients to be "weak-willed," "ugly," and "awkward."

These points were echoed in a forceful speech by Dr. William Bennett, coauthor of *The Dieter's Dilemma*. "Unlike most 'sick' people, who get some benefit from the presumption of innocence that goes with having a disease, fat people have been subjected to a guilt trip [for being] 'bad' patients," he said. And then added that, "This state of affairs has disastrous consequences for [their] health care, . . . Examinations may be done carelessly with the excuse that 'the fat gets in the way.' Symptoms may not be pursued and treatments may be half-heartedly offered with the thought, often unspoken, 'If he doesn't care about his health, why should I?' "

Unfortunately, Dr. Bennett's speech, which was given at a National Association to Advance Fat Acceptance (NAAFA) convention way back in 1982, seems to have fallen on deaf collegial ears.

The second ugly term that must be applied to many physicians is *igno-rance*, which causes them to fail their overweight patients in at least half a dozen ways:

First, they simply accept the premise that thinness is desirable for everyone, regardless of age or circumstances, and continue ordering their patients to diet—despite overwhelming evidence indicating that *all* diets have a 95–98 percent failure rate and are therefore useless at best and dangerously counterproductive at worst. And anyone who's been handed yet another badly photocopied sheet of yet another one-diet-fits-all scheme has seen this type of ignorance and indifference at first hand. Also, repeatedly receiving handfuls of the "freebie" diet pills that the most recent pharmaceutical smoothie dropped off at your doctor's office—followed by expensive prescriptions for that exact brand of pills—is equally disillusioning. Other physicians even exacerbate their patients' problems by restricting dietary carbohydrates so severely that muscle tissue and water are lost, but no body fat. And, of course, many of the more enterprising doctors have dreamed up their own diet "philosophies" and gone on to fortune and fame with best-sellers extolling such absurd propositions as inducing weight loss by eating all the carbohydrate-laden meat, cream, and cheese you can swallow (Dr. Robert Atkins); or consuming nothing but "protein-sparing" powder the doctor himself concocts, manufactures, and markets (Dr. Robert Linn).

Second, many physicians overlook the distinct possibility that their patients' conditions (such as elevated blood pressure, high cholesterol, heart and gallbladder maladies, and major depression) are caused, not by obesity, but by drastic and repeated weight loss efforts, and/or stress provoked by being the object of rampant societal prejudice. Yet proof of these possibilities began to be compiled and published in medical literature as long ago as 1983, when University of Toronto researchers Janet Polivy and C. Peter Herman published *Breaking the Diet Habit: The Natural Weight Alternative*. Their findings were corroborated in later studies by Harvard Medical School and the Michigan Department of Public Health.

Third, many doctors either remain oblivious to, or quarrel among themselves about, such critical research breakthroughs as the discovery of fat cells; the set-point theory; the relatively benign effect of excess weight on "pear-shaped" women (whose hips and legs are heavy), as opposed to those who are "apple-shaped" (with excess fat concentrated higher up); the "Cro-Magnon Catch-22," described in Chapter 3; and the fact that repeated dieting and consequent yo-yo weight levels are considered by many experts to be a significant health hazard that may shorten life expectancy—not to mention making permanent weight loss all but impossible. As for evolving *nutritional* theories regarding the treatment and prevention of obesity, to resort to the vernacular: Forget about it.

Fourth, doctors allow obesity to rage in epidemic proportions by rejecting every possible causation *except* patients' presumed overeating and laziness—even though several studies to the contrary have been widely publicized. Examples include an *American Journal of Clinical Nutrition* report in 1988, which proved that, on average, obese women actually eat less than thin women, just as they claim to; a study of identical twins at Quebec's Laval University by Dr. Claude Bouchard, indicating the strong influence of genetic heredity on weight levels; and various other data suggesting the strong possibility that obesity may be caused or exacerbated by heredity, food intolerances, insulin resistance, maladaptive brown adipose tissue, and other physical factors.

Fifth, they forget nature's decree that some degree of fatness is essential for women, especially for reproductive purposes. Examples of this reality, cited in "Rethinking Obesity," include preserving menstruation in young women (because, as most anorexics, some bulimics, and many fashion models and athletes have learned, when the level of body fat drops lower than approximately 15 percent, hormonal disruption can cause this monthly process to cease); reducing osteoporosis in older women (because severely limited body-fat levels can result in the loss of bone density); and lowering the incidence and severity of cancer and certain respiratory, infectious, and cardiovascular diseases. There has also been speculation that healthy people who *steadily* carry extra body weight may create the same strengthening effect on bones, joints, the heart, and other muscles that happens when bodybuilders strap on artificial weights during their workouts. I'm no scientist, but I consider myself living proof of this because my strength and stamina—for walking, swimming, and stair climbing, among other activities—often exceeds that of my thinner friends, and even my younger sister, who has always been slender.

And sixth, doctors who specialize in weight loss surgery do so in defiance of frightening research results indicating not only the potential danger of the operations themselves, which can multiply an obese patient's mortality risk ninefold, but the fact that the failure rate, in terms of weight loss, is as high as 75 percent. Additionally, some experts contend that every type of weight loss surgery carries the risk of at least two dozen different complications, including liver damage and severe malnutrition. Even more prevalent is uncontrollable life-long diarrhea.

I was lucky enough to have escaped these dire complications when I had my stomach stapled (yes, by the very surgeon recommended by the orthopedic doctor I consulted about my broken ankle). But the only permanent result of my gastroplasty is certainly not lasting weight loss; it's the permanent necessity of making myself throw up at least once a week, when food fails to "navigate" properly to its destination, either because of its texture, or because I haven't paid enough attention to the copious chewing that's necessary to prevent internal "gridlock" on the way down. And, I assure you, you haven't lived until you've had to induce vomiting in a public restroom at a restaurant, and then return to the dinner table trying to conceal your red face and watery eyes.

Worst of all is reflecting, at such times, on the fact that in my case, stomach stapling was an entirely inappropriate procedure. In the woefully rare instances when this type of surgery *does* work, it's generally because it averts voluminous eating, especially of dense food such as meat. Had my surgeon thought to interview me about my eating habits and preferences—rather than automatically presuming that my excess weight was caused by "standard" gluttony—he would probably have realized that, because I've never been a big eater and am practically a vegetarian, I was an unsuitable candidate. Thus, like the untold number of women whose situation resembles mine, I could have been spared undergoing a major operation, having an unsightly ten-inch scar on my midriff, and enduring a lifetime of being obliged to make myself throw up.

The third ugly term that must be applied to far too many physicians is
greed. Of course, the mother of all profit makers in this context is
weight loss surgery. Intestinal bypasses leapt from zero to 30,000 by
1980, and to 50,000 just two years later. For variety, there was the
insertion of gastric balloons, and stomach stapling. Although initially
mandated only for the "morbidly" obese (whose weight is at least 100
pounds more than "average"), before long it was full speed ahead and
damn the side effects and failure rates described above. Even women
with weights as low as 154 pounds have received the operations.

The most recent variation to come down the pike is so outrageous
that it drew cameras from *Prime Time Live* recently. Called the "Fibo
pouch procedure," after the surgeon who invented it, this operation
joins the esophagus to the small intestine. It bypasses the stomach
completely and relies on a tiny pocket at the end of the esophagus to
handle digestion—a chore for which nature never designed that organ.
Dr. Fibo admits that he has performed this operation on patients as
young as nine. And he says he has no doubts whatever about its efficacy, even when queried on camera about one of his patients, who had
developed so much scar tissue that she could no longer keep *any* food
down—and thus had to choose between death and a very tricky second operation to reverse her pouch procedure.

Why all the recklessness? It must have something to do with the
fact that the average cost for these surgical procedures is a whopping
$20,000. Multiplying that by the approximately 500 "bariatric" sur-
geons, who reportedly perform more than 50,000 operations throughout the country, reveals that this has become a billion-dollar industry.

When enthusiasm for weight loss surgery briefly flagged in the
1970s because of the failure rates and related deaths, along came liposuction (the mechanical sucking out of fat), which quickly became the
most frequently performed cosmetic operation in history. Complications, such as infections and lung embolisms from dislodged balls of
fat, gradually brushed some of the bloom off the rose. And then, in
the mid-1980s, after some twenty deaths occurred, not to mention
unsightly puckering, drawing, bumps, and unevenness for many of
those who survived, liposuction's popularity drooped. Whereupon
some genius promptly came up with modifications such as a smaller

fat-sucking tool (a cannula) and an equally refined new name: lipo-sculpturing.

Illustrating what a commonplace liposuction has become, sales and discount days are now being advertised—such as a recent one for the Zollman Center in Indianapolis, boasting, "27% Off Large Volume Liposuction." And a recent full-page ad for liposuction and other cosmetic surgery available at Jewish Hospital in Louisville, Kentucky, featured a photographically bloated "before" picture of Michelangelo's *David* beside an unretouched photo representing "after." What next? Two-for-one gastric balloons? Double-your-stomach-staples for one low, low price?

Collusion is another negative term that must be discussed in this context. What else can we call it when, every time the antifat profiteers dream up a cockamamie new scheme, thousands of physicians allow themselves to be courted, seduced, and kept in style by its marketers?

When some sadist came up with jaw wiring, for example, doctors stampeded to buy the necessary tools. When the absolute bonanza of human chorionic gonadotropin (HCG) injections came along, they had their patients literally lined up by the dozens every hour of the working day—and all it took was a minute or so with each one to weigh 'em, jab 'em, and head 'em out. Liquid protein fasts represented the same kind of labor-saving jackpot in that patients simply zipped in to their physicians' offices every week to be quickly weighed (usually by nurses) and sold another batch of expensive powder, and then zipped back out. Figuring in routine initial lab tests brought their total tab up to $54.75 for every pound (temporarily) lost on the protein-sparing regimen, according to a report published in *American Health*.

When metabolism-boosting amphetamine-laced diet drugs were all the rage, they were prescribed by the *billions*, despite such alarming side effects as strokes, heart damage, kidney failure, insomnia, anxiety, psychosis, and addiction. Eventually, these complications drew enough heat that the pills fell out of favor.

But in the early 1990s, new versions of "fat pills" once again began flooding the market. By far the most popular appetite suppressant is the "fen-phen" combination of fenfluramine and phentermine. Millions of prescriptions are now being written, despite the fact that fenfluramine is suspected of causing brain damage in monkeys and a related form, dexfenfluramine, was killing between twenty and forty women per year in France, and was under investigation there for causing seventy-eight cases of an incurable lung disease called primary pulmonary hypertension (PPH), until its restriction by French health officials in 1995.

Yet that same year, with fen-phen already in widespread use in this country—and reports of PPH, as well as mood alterations including depression and aggressiveness, trickling in from several states—the FDA approved a potent new related drug called Redux. It eventually will be available without prescription, both to commercial diet centers and directly to the public.

What's going on here? According to an alarming *Time* cover story, a worried majority of the FDA's advisory committee had at first refused to approve Redux. So the pro forces revisited the issue when they knew the anti's would be out of town at a convention. Result: The drug was approved by a one-vote margin. Arguments about its safety have raged ever since, but the approval stands, even in light of a report in the *New England Journal of Medicine* in the fall of 1996 which concluded that dexfenfluramine and similar diet drugs do indeed cause PPH, and that the risk soars by 3,000 percent when the pills are taken for longer than three months.

Nevertheless, publicity about Redux is driving millions of excited dieters to doctors' doors. The average monthly cost for Redux is about $114, not counting charges for examination and blood work. *Time* has reported that some 65,000 prescriptions per week are being written, making this "the fastest launch of any drug in the history of the pharmaceutical industry." Projections are that Redux will capture a $1 billion market share within five years.

Now are you ready for the kicker? Even while taking Redux, people *still* have to diet and exercise. And, while the drug does seem to help some people feel less hungry, their appetites return with a vengeance when they go off it. Some wonder drug!

Still another way for enterprising doctors to clean up is to use their medical credentials to get on the boards of big-bucks marketers—and in line for the gravy train of research grants. With a little luck, nobody will breathe the nasty words "conflict of interest." But somebody did when

National Association to Advance Fat Acceptance (NAAFA) executive director Sally E. Smith tipped over this rotten-apple cart in a hard-hitting piece in *USA Today* in 1995. She named several prominent physicians who frequently express prothinness opinions and—surprise! —just happen to be on the payroll of such antifat profiteers as Optifast and United Weight Control. Smith also reported that the ostensibly impartial 1991 conference of the North American Association for the Study of Obesity was actually funded by no fewer than eighteen diet-product and pharmaceutical biggies, including Jenny Craig, Weight Watchers, Nutri/System, Eli Lilly, Upjohn, and Hoffman/LaRoche.

As for psychotherapists, I doubt that Sigmund Freud ever modified his most famous question to "What do *fat* women want?" But if he were to travel from his time to ours and ask me to clue him in, I know exactly what I'd say: What we want, Herr Doktor, is simply respectful, informed, sincere help from those who followed in your footsteps.

It's certainly not what we're getting now. In fact, when troubled Fat Chicks are desperate enough to seek psychological lifelines, they frequently encounter the same sorts of disservice meted out by medical doctors. They ask and pay for help, but usually all they get are scorn and lectures, followed by tranquilizers, antidepressants, and diet sheets. Or years of expensive therapy aimed toward goals that are either impossible or reprehensible: lose enough weight to conform with society's unreasonable and unrealistic demands, or "adjust" to the role assigned them, which is basically two parts pariah to one part laughingstock. With the result—which bears repeating yet again—that eating disorders, depression, and general misery have reached epidemic proportions within the female population.

Who Else Is to Blame?

Research authorities, whose studies form the foundation for so much of the foregoing injustice, are also eminently blameworthy. We, the desperate public, are drowning in contradictory messages from clinical bozos who are evidently more interested in one-upping each other, and playing yet another round of Dueling Grant Proposals, than in buckling down to solving, or at least alleviating, the problems and the paradox of obesity. Rambunctious *Stop the Insanity* author Susan

Powter does a hilarious rap on this phenomenon to the effect that, every day, we're told something like: *Eat* lemons! And then the next day: *Don't* eat lemons!

We've all seen exactly this kind of argument ping-ponging through headlines about (to name only a few) margarine, oat bran, and pasta. And an even worse example of this sort of stalemating occurred when the National Institutes of Health first declared that yo-yo weight levels are lethally dangerous and, later, opined that they are not. This callous shilly-shallying about practices that have a significant impact on the health and lives of millions of women seems like unforgivable irresponsibility.

Why the miasma of confusion? To a great extent, it is due to the fact that many research studies are sponsored by companies (or whole industries) with financial stakes in the outcome of purportedly objective scientific investigations. Shocking examples cited by Cynthia Crossen in an eye-opening book titled *Tainted Truth: The Manipulation of Fact in America*, include a research report "proving" that white bread does not cause weight gain, a study that turned out to have been sponsored by the Wonder Bread company. Another equally outrageous report—to the effect that chocolate inhibits tooth decay—was funded by a dubious organization called the Princeton Dental Resource Center, which was financed by the candy company that manufactures M&Ms and Mars bars. And supposedly independent researchers, whose heralding of the wondrous effects of a thigh reduction cream triggered a $50,000 per day buying stampede, had actually pre-sold their formula to HerbaLife International, according to the *Tufts University Diet and Nutrition Letter*.

By the way, who do you think the FDA has put in charge of further clinical trials of Redux? Give up? Wyeth-Ayerst, the pharmaceutical company that manufactures the drug.

Even apart from the fox-guarding-the-henhouse factor, the contradictory messages that reach the public thanks to this double-dealing have resulted, to a dangerous extent, in a "What the hell" syndrome. It's a mental process by which we say to ourselves, consciously or subconsciously, "Hey, as long as nobody can manage to tell me conclusively what I should or shouldn't eat, what can I do but let myself off the hook and just do what I please? Might as well order up that double-cheese pizza with extra garlic butter. Who knows? Tomorrow, they might be saying *that's* what's good for us."

Bottom Line

I could go on and on about other ways in which physicians and other health professionals have failed to stop, or even denounce, the antifat propaganda machine—and instead have lent it legitimacy by going for the gold themselves. Instead, let's end this lengthy indictment by quoting some of the criticism that's beginning to be expressed about their mistreatment of overweight patients. The Institute of Medicine, for example, in a recent policy statement calling for "a fundamental change in public thinking about obesity," reported to Congress that "perhaps most lay persons, health care providers and even obese individuals themselves do not perceive the metabolic nature of the disease and thus view obesity as a problem of willful misconduct."

And concern about the epidemic levels of excess weight prompted Dr. William Dietz, director of clinical nutrition at the New England Medical Center in Boston, to take the extraordinary step of denouncing his colleagues in a recent op-ed piece in the *New York Times*. In it, he deplored the fact that "there is no commitment to obesity as a public health problem. We've ignored it, and blamed it on gluttony and sloth."

Yet another doctor, psychiatrist Theodore Isaac Rubin, broke ranks and defied collegial wrath two decades ago with this scorching indictment in *Alive and Fat and Thinning in America*: "There is an increasing number of so-called doctors who run weight-reduction mills and inflict on their innocent victims all kinds of extreme, fad, and inappropriate diets. [This] has become an ugly, multi-million-dollar business, both inside and outside the confines of established medicine."

But rather than obeying their Hippocratic oath to "first, do no harm," thousands of physicians have chosen instead to simply imitate the see-no-evil monkey. In so doing, they and their related health colleagues have allowed the antifat epidemic to rage out of control, while they cash in on their share of the billions spent by desperate people who've been convinced, beyond question, that—at all costs—they must be thin.

6

Hungry for Work

A nurturer of severely retarded children is denied work unless she loses weight. A lawyer quits her firm after being told too many times that clients "see her differently." A hotshot saleswoman can't get her foot in the door.

A nursing student is hounded out of school because she refuses to starve for her education. Flight attendants are grounded for fulfilling their chronological destiny. A policewoman is denied promotion for tipping weight scales her male colleagues don't even have to step onto. A health food clerk is rejected because slicing cheese, stocking shelves, and working the cash register are considered "too much" for her.

A talented editor who built an impressive resumé before her weight hit 200 is reduced to working as a typist in an out-of-sight work ghetto. A seventeen-year-old secretary, despite being well qualified, healthy, and energetic, is fired from her first job—at a life insurance company—because she weighs thirty pounds more than their mortality tables allow.

The most popular actress on a hit TV series is sacked because of her growing rotundity. The reigning Miss Universe is threatened with forced abdication if she doesn't knock off eighteen pounds in two weeks' time. The first female prime minister of Canada is a frequent target for vulgar potshots when she gains a bit of pudge.

....

If fat women really were as jolly as their reputation, they might see macabre humor in the absurdity of the *Too Fat Polka* that's been number one on the workplace charts ever since the billion-dollar brainwash began manipulating the attitudes of millions of people. But there's nothing funny about being literally forced to go hungry to obtain or retain a decent job. Or the fact that fully 60 percent of overweight North American women say they've been denied employment solely because of their appearance—or rather, because of prejudice against their appearance. And it's distinctly unhumorous that almost a third say that, when they do land jobs, they are routinely passed over for promotions and raises. Or that 78 percent say rampant cruelty and injustice have undermined their professional confidence. Or that they earn, on average, $6,700 less per year than thin women.

Extrapolating the percentages revealed in the most comprehensive survey ever done in this context—by NAAFA in 1987—means that at least 17 million American women are the victims of employment discrimination that is now illegal for every minority except the obese.

NAAFA's empirical proof came as no surprise to the legions of women affected by workplace discrimination. What *was* a shock was that the situation had become outrageous enough to land smack-dab on the front page of the *New York Times*. In what was undoubtedly the first time such respectful, high-caliber attention has been paid to the severity of what amounts to an epidemic of prejudice against the obese, the *Times* published a series called "Fat in America," which was written by Natalie Angier and Gina Kolata, and ran on page one for three days in November 1992.

There it all was, in sickening detail: Overweight workers are penalized one thousand dollars in salary for every "extra" pound. Obesity results in poverty for at least a third of women workers.* The vast majority of the overweight have been laughed at on the job and derided by fellow employees. Concluded Angier, "People who would

*By way of cruel contrast, the thinnest fashion models are paid the most money. Examples include Claudia Schiffer, who reportedly pulls in $5.3 million a year, and Kate Moss, who makes $2.2 million annually.

never publicly confess to racism have no qualms about expressing revulsion for the obese."

Two years later, *USA Today* ran a front-page story about similar findings by a British study of 12,536 schoolchildren who were followed from the late 1950s to the present. "It seems," said an accompanying commentary by Dr. Catherine DeAngelis, "that it's over for the 'fat lady' long before she sings." Adds Dr. Susan C. Wooley, director of the eating-disorders clinic at the University of Cincinnati, "We're running out of people that we're allowed to hate and to feel superior to. Fatness is the one thing left that seems to be a person's fault—which it isn't."

The commendable *New York Times* series, and publicity about the British study, were balm for many a broken heart and extended temporary dignity to many a reviled antifat victim. But they weren't enough of an eye-opener to make a difference. Name an industry—from high finance to health care, aviation, electronics, communications, law, and even law enforcement—and you'll find abuse. Sometimes the abuse takes the form of bare-faced prejudice. Sometimes it appears in the form of flimsy smoke screens based on fallacious health-insurance rationales. And sometimes it's just so ludicrous it defies analysis. Or, rather, it begs the question answered by Robert F. Murphy's *The Body Silent*. This moving book examines the prejudicial atmosphere in which a group whose oppression parallels that of the obese is forced to exist: "The disabled serve as constant, visible reminders to the able-bodied that the society they live in is a counterfeit paradise, that they too are vulnerable. We represent a fearsome possibility."

Top of the Heap

It's hard to imagine more odious evidence of antifat bias than what turned up in a recent attitudinal survey of 1,139 top-level CEOs, presidents, and executive vice presidents—none of whom were overweight. The results clearly demonstrate that both halves of the "lean and mean" metaphor have been transmuted into literal reality by the folks at the top. Epitomizing the overall tone was this nasty remark from Donald Lennox, former CEO of Navistar International Transportation: "I don't like fat people. If I were recruiting and some guy waddled in with a big gut, he'd be dead before he opened his mouth."

And a fat female candidate would be unlikely to get an opportunity to "waddle" into Mr. Lennox's august presence, according to University of Pittsburgh psychology professor Dr. Irene Frieze. "Grossly overweight females are penalized more severely than men with the same problem," she concluded upon completing a study of 1,200 MBA graduates for her university. Results for the males: Upper-level managers who are 20 percent overweight earn approximately $4,000 a year less than their average-weight counterparts. Results for the 350 female MBAs: nonexistent—there were too few fat women in top management to be statistically significant!

"Bosses interpret weight gain in a woman employee," said Frieze, "as a signal that she's abandoned any hope of rising higher." Of course, the fallacy in that "interpretation"—though the bosses would doubtless deny it—precisely parallels what George Bernard Shaw said long ago in a similar context: "The American white relegates the black to the rank of shoeshine boy and then concludes that the black is good for nothing but shining shoes."

Summing up the attitudes toward obesity among powerful and influential executives, psychologist Leonard J. Donk, a California counselor to Fortune 500 companies, says, "The profundity of the narrow-mindedness is incredible." To which Lynn Smith, president and CEO of St. Louis's Dunhill Personnel, adds, "I've had employers say to me, only half-jokingly, 'Can't you find us someone who's blond, blue-eyed, and has a flat stomach?' "

The picture gets no brighter as you climb down the corporate ladder or venture farther from the mega-power bases.

Sales

Take what happened to saleswoman Diane Wildowsky when she weighed 230 pounds. Granted, her profession is one of the most notoriously image-conscious. But with a successful track record in cutthroat New York City, she thought she'd be a shoo-in as a representative for an apparel company in the Northwest. "Over the phone, they liked everything they heard," she recalls. But in her face-to-face interview, Wildowsky was "stunned. Here he was trying to get me out of his office. I was never even considered."

The product was large-size women's clothing.

But even this degree of self-defeating executive stupidity is standard practice in sales, according to personnel authorities. "Anyone who's supposed to meet with customers and is more than forty pounds over-weight is going to have a big-time problem," says Connecticut-based Peter Floyd, of Personnel Corporation of America. "Managers assume that overweight people don't have the energy or drive to operate in the field as salespersons," adds Chicago outplacement executive James E. Challenger. "Not only is it harder for fat people to get jobs, they tend to lose them faster."

These assessments are amplified by a recent study of the effects of obesity on service careers, such as sales, done by Professor Michael L. Klassen, of the University of Northern Iowa. The overweight, he found, are considered (in rank order): "lazy, unkempt, jolly, lacking self-discipline, lacking self-care, unhealthy, and insecure."

And, says Martin Everett, general editor of *Sales & Marketing Management*, the crowning irony of the fact that "most sales executives won't look twice at a fat candidate" is that the bias is flourishing "despite mounting difficulty in finding field sales talent."

Law

No eye-popping studies such as Klassen's have been done of the legal profession, probably because discretion is the bedrock for attorneys. So it's not surprising that, even though the American Bar Association *Journal* and several other professional publications have reported that disenchanted female attorneys are quitting the law in droves, only one has gone public about what it's like to be an overweight lady lawyer.

"All fat people are 'outed' by their appearance," wrote Buffalo, New York, attorney Jennifer A. Coleman in a recent *Newsweek* "My Turn" column. "But . . . I really believed I could infiltrate the ranks of the non-fat and thereby establish my worth . . . by a regimen of swimming, cycling and jogging that put all but the most compulsive to shame. I ate only cottage cheese, brown rice, fake butter and steamed everything . . ." Coleman's weight didn't budge, and, "fit but still fat," she queried, "How was it I was still lazy, weak, despised, a slug and a cow? I finally real-ized: It didn't matter what I did. I was and always would be the object

of sport, derision, antipathy and hostility so long as I stayed in my body."
So, after hearing much too often the veiled insult from superiors at the
large firms for which she had always worked that "clients looked at me
differently," Coleman told me she'd decided to become a sole practitioner. Her new specialty: employment discrimination.

To be scrupulously fair, however, is it possible that what appear to be
straightforward cases of size discrimination are actually hardheaded
business decisions? In some cases, the deplorable but true answer is
yes. A study of business students, for example, shows that, when they
are customers, they flat out hate being served by overweight people
(of both genders). Does this justify not hiring the obese? Social commentator Lindsy Van Gelder has this eloquent answer: "If a business
claimed that it needed to discriminate against Jewish workers in order
to protect its image with its anti-Semitic customers, no one would suggest religious conversion as a solution to the problem. But an 'unattractive' job applicant? The onus instantly switches to what she should
do to 'fix' herself."

Which brings us to the broader context in which employment discrimination against Fat Chicks flourishes. It's actually just the latest
chapter in a very old story: backlash against the emancipation of women.
In the all-too-recent past, the male powers-that-be fought tooth and nail
to keep women out of their exclusive domain—the workplace. When
the battle was lost, at least from the point of view of the most dim-
witted "old boys," a cunning way was found either to disqualify the
female usurper at the starting-gate or to undermine her success and
self-confidence when she did land a job. The new deal: whatever the
position, the prerequisite for females would be attractiveness. Why? As
Naomi Wolf expresses it in *The Beauty Myth*: "Employers did not simply develop the beauty backlash because they wanted office decora-
tion. . . . [the] triumph of 'beauty' ideologies . . . came about as a result
of real fear on the part of the central institutions of our society about
what might happen if free women made free progress in free bodies
throughout a system that calls itself a meritocracy."

So, to ensure that the hordes of women flooding the workplace
were anything but free to threaten the existing power structure, what
Wolf calls a "third shift" was added. Women would now be coerced

into a daily grind of not just one professional shift, as men have, and not just the two they had already been holding down at home and at work, but also a third shift, which consisted of maintaining a standard of appearance that had previously been demanded only of professional beauties, such as models and actresses.

Thus was born the concept of jobs as never-ending beauty contests—a notion whose ludicrousness becomes instantly obvious if it's applied to men. But the fact is, we don't perceive the third shift as the added burden that it is. Women—aided and abetted by many of the same profiteers who convinced everyone that "fat" equals "ugly"—fell for the self-defeating ruse hook, line, and sinker.

Now, rather than insisting that their worthiness be judged solely by the official BFOQ—bona fide occupational qualification—rule that was established in the name of equal opportunity, as Wolf writes, "women . . . are persuaded to trim their desires and self-esteem neatly into the discriminatory requirements of the workplace, while putting the blame for the system's failures on themselves alone."

Blimpos Anonymous

That induced sense of self-blame ran like a disturbing undercurrent beneath the tales recounted during a recent meeting of an all-woman obesity support group in a small Midwestern city. Like children feigning courage by whistling past the graveyard, these women call their group Blimpos.

"If you can see the humor and the defiance in that name," explained the group's founder, "then you're ready for Blimpos." Tess* then called for someone to kick off what she called a "moan and groan" session, devoted, on this occasion, to employment experiences.

Tugging her thigh-length shirt away from her hips and stomach, in a defensive gesture that's second nature to large women, Daisy steps to the front of the room. "I'd like to frame my comments tonight into a literary context," she says, in a quietly defiant voice. "As some of you know, I had a damn good career going as a magazine editor when I was slim. And now all I can get is word processing, at a third of my

*The names used here are pseudonyms.

former salary. Well, this is how Virginia Woolf described the psychological effect of that kind of squashing in *A Room of One's Own*:
"always to be doing work that one did not wish to do, and to do it like
a slave . . . and then the thought of that one gift which it was death to
hide . . . perishing and with it my self, my soul. . . .' "

There's a smattering of applause. And then a voice from the side of
the room. "I know exactly what you mean," says Gillian. "I'm holding
on to my crummy job as a factory assembler because I'm a realist, but
I feel like I'm just withering. Whenever I read the classifieds, all I see
are companies that wouldn't even let me in the door. Anything to do
with food, forget it. They'd see me as a walking advertisement why
customers shouldn't buy their product. And ditto for anything that's
based on image—like sales or receptionist."

"Aw, come on," objects Annie from the other side of the room. "What
isn't considered an image job these days?" After an explosion of affir-
mative responses, Tess asks for specific examples of job discrimination.

Ginny recalls the division of labor when she worked in the ad section of a publication. "Only the thin women were allowed to go out
and make cold calls, and of course, that's where the big commissions
are. All the overweight girls were kept in the office on lowly telephone sales."

"Sure, and how about me?" queries Katie. "I've been working with
an employment agency for months now, looking for something in desk-
top publishing. My counselor says, if anything, I'm overqualified and
any employer would be lucky to get me. But she hasn't sent me on any
interviews in the last two months. When I asked her why, she got all
embarrassed. Then she sort of whispered, 'I know I shouldn't tell you
this because I could get in trouble. But the last place I sent you, that
advertising agency, told me they'd snap you up in a minute—if you
weighed fifty pounds less.' "

"Yeah," says Nancy. "They've even got a code for that. If they write
'NFO' on your file, it means 'Not Front Office.' In other words, they
won't even bother sending you on interviews unless your appearance
is up to snuff. And we know what that means, don't we?"

"Well, I've tried and tried to talk myself out of believing this,"
muses Shannon. "But when I had a great job as a paralegal, I ended
up making a very bad enemy. He obviously felt that I should be obse-

quious and apologetic just because I was fat. I reported him [to upper management], but eventually it got so bad that I felt I had to quit. They had to assign, literally, three and a half people to do what I had been doing. But when the creep left a few months later and I tried to get my job back, they wouldn't even take my calls. I know I was good at what I did, so what reason other than prejudice could they have for just letting me go like that, even when it costs them big bucks?"

"Just about the same thing is happening to me right now," adds Paula. "I know I'm excellent at what I do and I've worked like a maniac to get where I am. So I try to behave like the other people at my management level, you know, like I expected to be respected and listened to. But it's just not happening. It's as if everybody's demanding that I act like some kind of fool, and then they get furious when I don't."

"But it isn't just about getting a job," pipes up a younger woman named Chris. "It's also about what it's like every day at work if you're overweight. This might sound picayune but there's this manager who always comes into my department with donuts for everybody. And almost every day he says something at the top of his voice about how I really shouldn't have one. I never do, but people keep laughing, so he keeps on saying it."

Rejoinders come flying from all over the room. "I was sexually harassed for over a year until I finally quit. But, to this day, nobody believes it could have happened just because of the way I look."

"Three of us who are overweight were the constant butt of jokes everywhere we went in the plant, and one day in the cafeteria, some jerks actually threw food at us. But the union wouldn't do a thing."

"My company now has a really good program to help people with alcohol or drug problems. They don't even lose pay or seniority when they go to dry out. But fat is supposed to be your own fault, so all you ever get is grief for being a lazy, disgusting slob."

See You in Court?

None of the women described so far has chosen to take her justifiable grievances to court. Maybe it's because the brave women who *have* done so have experienced decidedly mixed results.

Elder Care: An example of the inescapable Catch-22 trap that permeates weight discrimination cases snared a Michigan nurse's aide in the case of Krein v. Marian Manor Nursing Home. After satisfactorily tending to the nursing home's elderly patients for five years, Melanie Krein was fired because of her obesity. She attempted to sue Marian Manor, but the suit was dismissed by the trial court. When Krein appealed, the state supreme court concurred with the lower court that "the mere assertion that one is overweight or obese is not enough to make a person a member of a protected class."

Translation: Most American courts maintain that obesity is not a disqualification, and therefore is not covered by human rights safeguards for minorities. But employers who wish to contend that obesity *is* a disqualification are completely free to fire, refuse to hire, or professionally squelch overweight workers.

Mental Health Care: Even in a case where the clients couldn't possibly be presumed to have antifat sentiments, a large woman can experience employment discrimination. For five years, Bonnie Cook had satisfactorily performed her work as an aide at a Rhode Island residential center for severely retarded children. Her daughter's illness forced her to resign for a time, and when she reapplied for her former position, she was refused it because of her 320-pound weight.

When Cook sued the state Department of Mental Health, Retardation and Hospitals, Dr. Mark O'Brien testified that he had turned her down because her "morbid obesity" made her "susceptible" to a host of health problems. But the doctor's hypothesis was shattered by the fact that Cook's weight was exactly the same when she reapplied as it had been when she was considered a satisfactory employee.

In the first such victory in an American federal appeals court, Cook won her job back, plus retroactive pay and seniority, and $100,000 in punitive damages. Says Rhode Island Civil Liberties Union executive director Steve Brown, "The irony of this is that we have an agency that has worked hard to change public attitudes toward the mentally disabled, and here they are discriminating against someone based on all the stereotypes of obesity." Echoes Cook herself, "All I can say is that people shouldn't judge others because of how they look. What's important is whether or not they can do the job."

Retail Clerking: Across the continent, in Santa Cruz, California, Toni Cassista applied for a clerking job at a health food store called Community Foods. When she got the old don't-call-us routine and later saw the job readvertised, she launched a one-woman counterattack that eventually grew into a statewide cause célèbre.

"I started small," she recalls, "by simply asking why I wasn't hired." The response was that "a fat person could not work on [her] feet eight hours a day, forty hours a week, and that slicing cheese, working the cash register, or stocking shelves would be too much for me." Knowing that the employee-owned health food store had a progressive reputation, Cassista first tried sweet reason, trying to raise store personnel's consciousness about size-diversity issues. When they turned a deaf ear, she filed a complaint with the California Department of Fair Employment and Housing.

Community Foods then offered to settle out of court, but Cassista refused. "This is not about money," she insisted. "Everything that I am—my self-worth, my self-respect, and my dignity—[is] at stake. Employers need to get a strong message that any applicant who walks through the door should be treated equally . . . that if certain physical abilities are necessary to do the job, a test of those abilities should be incorporated into the hiring process."

Cassista eventually won what so far is a purely Pyrrhic victory. The California court that heard her case made legal history when it decreed that the burden of proof in employment discrimination cases should shift from the plaintiff to the defendant. If the state supreme court concurs, Cassista and Community Foods will head back to the courtroom. But this time, the health food store will have to prove it didn't discriminate, rather than Cassista having to show the opposite.

At the federal level, however, the situation was made gloomier for all categories of job discrimination plaintiffs in 1993. Two years earlier, in what the *Los Angeles Times* and others called "a clear slap at the high court," Congress enacted an amendment to the Civil Rights Act to make it easier for mistreated employees to pursue employment discrimination cases. It also made them eligible to have jury trials and to claim damages. But the U.S. Supreme Court tipped the teeter-totter once again by upholding the "reverse onus" situation that places upon plaintiffs, rather than defendants, the burden of proving that bias was the cause of their dismissal.

Incidentally, while the Cassista case was in the spotlight in Santa Cruz, California's first public forum on appearance discrimination was staged there. Spearheaded by NAAFA and the city's Human Rights Task Force, the debate drew national attention to what boors delighted in calling "a freak show." On one side were proponents of size acceptance such as Michael Coonerty, who stated, "Appearance discrimination cripples businesses because they aren't hiring the best qualified people. They are hiring for ridiculous, unrealistic reasons."

On the opposite side was chief opponent Louise Rittenhouse, who snarled, "If [the antidiscrimination ordinance passes] and I have two equally qualified candidates for employment, one thin and well dressed [and] the other obese and dirty ... I have to discriminate against the thin, clean one or I go to court."

When the ordinance did pass, influential media pundit Rush Limbaugh—a three-hundred-pounder who apparently misunderstands the nature of glass houses—cast a characteristically insensitive stone. "I want an ordinance," he sarcastically thundered from his radio-bully pulpit, "prohibiting ugly people from walking on city streets during daylight hours."

Law Enforcement: Since there are so few laws protecting the overweight, it's not surprising that even law enforcement workers can be tagged for obesity. In the California case of Donoghue v. County of Orange, a female police department clerk decided to train for a deputy sheriff position. Carole Donoghue underwent the same boot-camp conditions as the male candidates. But the daily weigh-ins were mandatory only for her and for the one other woman in the program. After incurring repeated reprimands for exceeding the women-only weight limit, she was ultimately terminated.

Donoghue filed a complaint with the Equal Employment Opportunity Commission (EEOC), which found in her favor, concluding that males who were even more overweight than she were not punished or penalized, let alone terminated. She also prevailed at trial on the grounds that her civil rights had been violated. It's important to note, however, that this case was essentially a victory against sexual, rather than weight, discrimination.

Jury Duty: At least one officer of the court does whatever he can to keep overweight women off his juries. San Diego deputy district attorney August Meyer was recently quoted in the *San Diego Union* as contending that not only does it take a man "to make the tough decisions," but the obese "don't have the sort of social contact and work-together skills of someone I would like to [have] on my jury. They tend to be outcasts and unhappy people."

The Military: As the military looks for ways to trim ranks now that the Cold War is over, a quiet little "police action" is being waged against overweight personnel. The experience of Nyleen Mullally, who had served for thirteen years with the Minnesota National Guard, is typical. Without warning, she says, she was suddenly chewed out by her commander for "getting away with" excessive weight for too long. He froze her advancement for three years of what she calls "hell" until she resigned. Eight months later, as if in an attempt to place one final blow, Mullally was, she says, "called to involuntary active duty in Operation Desert Storm. The war was short and I was discharged [without going to the Middle East], but I was never weighed. I was just told that the weight standards had been 'waived' for the duration."

Nursing: Sharon Russell is an overweight woman whose professional problems, and exemplar status, were dramatic enough to interest even *60 Minutes* and *People.* Now a successful nurse in Florida, she was nearly prevented from getting her RN because of size discrimination. Russell, while an A student at Rhode Island's Salve Regina College, was expelled for failing to comply with an edict to lose two of her approximately three hundred pounds every week. Why the career-threatening ultimatum? Because school administrators ostensibly feared she would "lack credibility" in counseling patients on the subject of nutrition.

Russell completed her nursing degree elsewhere and sued Salve Regina for breach of contract. She won a $44,000 award at the first trial, based on a judgment that she had been dismissed "because she was obese and for no other reason." But the school, whose lawyer put forward the non sequitur "I don't know of any blind people who are nurses [and] doctors don't write charts in Braille," appealed all the way to the U.S. Supreme Court. There, on a jurisdictional technicality, Russell's victory was overturned and sent down to the First Circuit Court in Boston, where it is still stalled as of this writing.

Aviation: Another category of well-publicized court cases involved thousands of women who weigh far less than Sharon Russell, but whose careers were even more jeopardized by weight gains. The flight attendants of American Airlines, Pan American, United, USAir, and Delta fought plucky and protracted battles to get punitive weight policies rescinded. Not until federal EEOC attorneys entered the fray did the hostility in the so-called friendly skies toward aging and thickening flight attendants grab the spotlight.

Even now, when those loathsome "Fly Me" slogans have been jettisoned, the employment manual of, for example, American Airlines still states that "a firm, trim silhouette, free of bulges, rolls, or paunches, is necessary for an alert, efficient image." But, countered the EEOC, women who don't gain some weight as they pass age forty risk health problems.

The parting shots in the fracas have gone to a variety of judges over the past few years. Pan Am was ordered to pay $2.35 million to 116 female flight attendants and to reinstate those who had been fired. Chided Judge Thelton E. Henderson, "The Court finds Pan Am's weight policy perpetuated a sexual stereotype that female flight attendants must be slim-bodied, attractive women, rather than competent employees."

Succumbing to the "Weigh my performance, not my body" rallying cry of furious flight attendants, American Airlines relaxed its archaic weight restrictions to an allowable maximum of 145 (up from 129) pounds for flight attendants aged forty to forty-four. And both Delta and USAir stopped weigh-ins for flight attendants altogether. Yet insiders predict that, though this particular battle was won, the war may yet resume because the industry still considers alluring flight attendants a vital part of its competitive stock in trade.

Entertainment: So far, there have been only a few spotlighted cases of weight discrimination in Hollywood, but—probably because so many people think slenderness is automatically a BFOQ for actresses—none had the sort of "Anita Hill effect" that I believe will one day begin turning the situation around. Delta Burke, who played Suzanne Sugarbaker, the most popular character on the *Designing Women* TV series, was hounded about her escalating weight by her producers, humiliated in the press, and ultimately fired. Three years later, however, secret behind-the-scenes negotiations created a new role for Burke. With what looked like every one of her "extra" pounds intact, she went on to star as a congresswoman on *Women of the House*—a comedy series that was developed by Linda Bloodworth-Thomason and her husband, the same duo who had previously sacked Burke.

Kathy Bates, the only large woman ever to win a best-actress Oscar (for *Misery*),* was denied the movie version of her Broadway success in *Frankie and Johnny*. Instead, the role of the depressed, down-at-the-heels waitress went to the least logical candidate—glamorous, rail-thin Michelle Pfeiffer. Actually, Bates was accustomed to this process by then, because she'd also been passed over for the film versions of two of her other stage triumphs: *'Night Mother* and *Crimes of the Heart*, which went to reed-slender Sissy Spacek and Diane Keaton.

More recently, actress Janeane Garofalo was amazingly candid about what it took to land a starring role in the film *The Truth About Cats and Dogs*: losing 35 pounds. Nothing too unusual about that in show-biz, right? But Garofalo's premovie weight was only 140 pounds. And the character she played is called an "ugly bitch," and considers herself so unattractive that she can't bring herself to reveal her identity to the man she loves, instead coaxing a skinny model to stand in for her. Hollywood's "imagery of the 'plain' person," says Garofalo, "is galling. I don't feel I've done the right thing, [and] I don't condone what I've done. It's just a reality . . ."

And how about Miss Universe? Well, thanks to strict dieting and working out three hours a day, Alicia Machado had whipped her five-foot, seven-inch frame down to 112 pounds just in time to enter the

---

*Portly Hattie McDaniel won a best supporting actress Oscar for 1938's *Gone With the Wind*.

1996 international beauty pageant. She won. But, rather than trilling platitudes about working for world peace, the Venezuelan teenager surprised the watching world by vowing to "eat, eat, eat and sleep."

Result: Machado "ballooned" up to 130 pounds, whereupon irate pageant authorities reportedly demanded that she shrink back down to her victory weight in a mere two weeks, before her next major appearance. After news of the incident exploded in the world press (sample headline: "The Beauty and the Beastly Weightwatchers"), the officials backed down (and denied everything). But the pressure was revived when entrepreneur extraordinaire Donald Trump bought the Miss Universe franchise. He called Machado "an eating machine," declared that "the crown comes with absolute obligations," and ordered her to embark on a very public reducing regimen.

Electronics Technology: One of the few cases in which the irresistible force of justice has met the immovable object of prejudice—and the object moved—occurred in the vital field of electronics technology. It took ten tenacious years, with setbacks every step of the way, but Catherine McDermott ultimately trounced the mighty Xerox Corporation.

After succeeding in similar positions elsewhere, the 249-pound systems consultant had been hired by Xerox. But she flunked the pre-employment physical solely, as she proved in court, because of her weight. Xerox, which submitted no evidence that McDermott's size was an impediment to her work performance, was ordered by the New York State human rights board to hire her, with equivalent back pay.

But that decision was overturned on appeal by the same application of Catch-22 reasoning that defeated Melanie Krein: Since McDermott had proven that she was not disabled, her obesity was deemed a "voluntary condition," and therefore she was not among the groups whose human rights are protected in the context of employment. Of McDermott's later victory in a higher court, the *Labor Law Journal* remarked, "It is significant to note that Xerox forthrightly claimed that nothing was wrong with her, but that it was concerned about the 'potential' impairments she might develop in the future. Similar concerns have been increasingly voiced by other companies [which] see people like McDermott . . . as a burden."

Health Insurance—No Laughing Matter

Isn't it funny how such burdensome "potential impairment" scenarios apply only to the Catherine McDermotts, and not to, say, bungee-jumpers, motorcyclists, hot-air-balloon enthusiasts, or even smokers, all of whom incur health risks far more voluntarily than do the obese?

The *Labor Law Journal* hit the health insurance nail squarely on its head in characterizing one of the earliest lawsuits in the context of weight discrimination as merely "the first red flag that signaled the interest of employers in having an . . . illness-free and claim-free labor force . . ." NAAFA cofounder William J. Fabrey agrees with that, but adds that "all too often, the employer's real reason for not wanting to hire fat job applants lies in the area of aesthetics—they feel the fat person would be bad for the corporate image."

Nevertheless, the crisis of mushrooming health-care costs is certainly no laughing matter, and the legitimate health consequences for any employee group—the overweight included—cannot simply be disregarded. At this writing, the rules of the American health insurance game are being vociferously debated. Whatever the outcome, what probably will never change is the employers' right to establish general eligibility standards for the health insurance coverage they provide.

Overweight workers essentially have no problem with that, nor with the legitimate implementation of "wellness" programs. At least not so long as the criteria applied to them are as fair as those applied to other workers, and are not just knee-jerk, prejudicial assumptions about their capabilities and the amount of money they might cost in health insurance claims. Currently, however, as pioneering obesity specialist Dr. Albert Stunkard, of the University of Pennsylvania, told the *New York Times* for the "Fat in America" series: "The extent to which overweight people have difficulty in obtaining work goes far beyond what can be justified by medical data and must be due to discrimination."

A striking case in point was provided in 1995, when the first jury ever to go this far financially awarded an obese San Francisco man $1 million in damages. Pundits everywhere hooted when they heard that John Rossi had been fired by an auto parts store because he weighed four hundred pounds. What most of them didn't hear—or didn't acknowledge—was that Rossi had held the job from which he was fired for ten years, and had taken a grand total of three sick days in all that time.

Shades of Things to Come?

Keeping all of the above in mind, consider how much outrage would explode in this country if a high-profile corporation began docking five dollars per paycheck from all workers who were, say, Democrats, or whose spouses were Democrats—until they stopped being Democrats.

Substitute the word "fat" for "Democrats" and you've got the exact situation that U-Haul International recently began imposing on its workforce. Some 13,500 employees were required to sign statements swearing that they, *and* their spouses, would either comply with the company's so-called wellness weight level or consent to a salary reduction. The penalty for lying: immediate dismissal.

U-Haul's policy scarcely made a news ripple, even though the American Civil Liberties Union denounced it as "barbaric . . . unconscionable [and] outrageous." But corporate bean counters were paying attention, and not just to U-Haul's punitive ploy, which conceivably could chop $250,000 off the company's annual salary expenses. Beady-eyed bottom-liners also evidently noticed the national indifference toward oppression of the obese. And now authorities such as the *Labor Law Journal* predict that "more than half of the major corporations will [soon] implement such programs [as U-Haul's]."

Yet companies who find U-Haul's example enticing would do well to think about the broader implications. For sheer practicality, employee policies must be considered from the perspective that more than one-third of the American population—including the available labor pool—is now at least 20 percent overweight, while millions of others are even heavier, and overall obesity has been on the rise for the past few decades.

Add to that the calculation by the Census Bureau that, for the next seventeen years, an American will turn fifty every 7.5 seconds. By the turn of the century, the members of this age group—known *ad infinitum* as the baby boomers—will number in excess of 80 million. This will make them the biggest—in both senses of the word—demographic group of all. The boomers' economic and sociological clout has already enabled its members to rewrite the social contract in many significant ways. In the context of employment, it seems entirely predictable that, both as workers and as consumers, they will demand a new definition of "normality."

To illustrate the point, two giant companies serve as perfect examples of how abstemious employee policies would decimate profits if adopted as general business practices. Coors workers and their counterparts at Hershey now know that if they chug enough of their employer's beer or munch enough of its chocolate bars to sprout soft flab, they'll pay for it in hard cash.

At Hershey, 650 nonunion employees were recently ordered to report to a health-screening site to be weighed, measured, and quizzed about their diet and exercise habits. Those found "least fit" stand to lose $1,404 per year in company health benefits. Similarly, at Coors, only those employees who meet management's "wellness" standards are eligible to have 90 percent of their medical bills covered by the company-subsidized health insurance plan.

But don't expect to see this Big Brotherly attitude creeping into either of these companies' advertisements any time soon. Consumers will be encouraged, to the tune of millions of ad dollars, to keep eating and drinking without regard for the consequences.

Another comestibles corporation, Stouffer Foods, was the target of what is thought to be the first class-action suit ever brought by overweight workers in North America. But this time it was management that had to dig into its pockets because of strict antifat policies. In 1993, Stouffer's parent company, Nestlé, was forced to settle out of court with fifty-one obese job applicants who had filed a federal discrimination suit after being turned down because of their weight. The company ended up paying a plump $303,000 to forty-five of the overweight complainants and hiring six of those it had previously rejected.

Unfortunately, the suit's potential fizzled, both as a legal precedent and in terms of publicity, because it never went to court, and also because the claims of the obese applicants were rolled in with those of a larger group of racial-minority workers who had also been turned away by Stouffer.

Is Legislation the Answer?

For all intents and purposes, weight discrimination is simply not against the law at the federal level and in thirty-nine states. In eleven other states, light has been glimpsed at the end of the tunnel, with either the enactment or the introduction of legislative antidotes to the antifat plague spread by the billion-dollar brainwash. These include California, Colorado, Illinois, Maryland, Michigan, Nevada, New York, North Dakota, Rhode Island, Tennessee, and Texas.

Michigan led the way with its sweeping Elliott-Larsen Civil Rights Act of 1977. The pioneering legislation decreed that "an employer shall not: fail or refuse to hire, or recruit, or discharge, or otherwise discriminate against an individual with respect to employment, compensation, or a term, condition, or privilege of employment, because of religion, race, color, national origin, age, sex, height, weight or marital status."

It took New York State sixteen years to catch up with Michigan. But Bill A.3484, which was proposed by Assemblyman Daniel Feldman in the spring of 1993, is now being touted as a model for other jurisdictions. Feldman persevered despite ridicule from (among many others) the generally compassionate Mario Cuomo, then governor of New York, who publicly called the proposal "one law too many."

Feldman responded by appearing at a press conference called by NAAFA to endorse and publicize his bill. "For too many years, people have experienced blatant prejudice because of size," said Feldman. "This may be the last form of discrimination that conventional thinking accepts—but that acceptance must be ended." Added NAAFA executive director Sally E. Smith: "We are a society that prides itself on equal opportunity for all and a society that likes to believe that anyone can reach for the American dream. Assemblyman Feldman's bill will go far to ensure that this dream is available to all people, regardless of body size."

As the New York antidiscrimination act awaits passage, the overweight there and elsewhere remain as vulnerable as were women and racial minorities until the advent of equal-opportunity employment policies and sharp-toothed laws to back them up. Unless and until that scenario is extended to the obese, say legal authorities, there is only one legislative umbrella to shelter them from the storm of prejudice: the federal Americans with Disabilities Act (ADA).

Until passage of the laudable ADA in 1992, employers were as free to ignore and exploit the disabled as they still are with regard to the obese. Now, however, it's a whole new ball game for the physically challenged, with Uncle Sam acting as a stern umpire. In essence, the ADA legally protects the disabled from any employment discrimination that isn't based solely on reasonable job-related qualifications. That, of course, is all the disabled, the overweight, or indeed any other workers, need ask.

So, in light of scientific data indicating that as much as 70 percent of obesity may be genetically caused, some see the ADA as legal salvation for the overweight in employment, housing, and many other contexts. Says attorney Jennifer Coleman, "It is my conviction that obesity is a clinical condition, not a moral fault. And that's exactly what the ADA is all about." A recent article in the *Labor Law Journal* concurred with her: "Protecting the obese, who suffer discrimination due to untrue stereotypes, conforms with [the] legislative intent."

In practical terms, and in the absence of specific protective legislation for the obese, both of these opinions are correct. But if ever the term "double-edged sword" had a perfect application, this is it. If Fat Chicks accept the protection of the ADA, or any future human-rights legislation based on disability, they must—by definition—accept being defined as "disabled." But the truth is that, for all but the truly huge, and for almost all job categories, extra weight is not disabling.

Bonnie Cook satisfactorily tended the retarded children in her care for five years, despite weighing 320 pounds. Toni Cassista would gladly have accepted a mandatory probation period in which to prove whether she could function efficiently in the health food store that refused to hire her. Kim Campbell's performance as prime minister was not affected in the slightest by her modest weight gain. And that teenage secretary who was fired from her first job—whose name was Terry Poulton—could surely have managed to type, file, and take dictation without dropping dead because of thirty extra pounds.*

---

*I might add that simply believing obesity disqualified me from topflight employment prevented me from becoming a journalist until I was well past thirty. Ironically, I've since realized that I had been an accomplished writer as a little girl. The point is, if you're convinced you're barred from any goal, you will not pursue it, no matter what your abilities. And it goes without saying that a profound lack of encouragement to do so will worsen the situation.

The fact is, whatever incapacity pertains in most employment discrimination situations—be it weight, disability, sex, or race—is literally in the eye of the beholder. Yet, even for her own protection, we would scarcely think of applying a "disabled" label to, say, a Native American who lost an employment opportunity because of prejudice. Labels—particularly those that diminish and are not genuinely applicable—are the problem for Fat Chicks, not the solution.

What *would* be fair and effective? In my opinion, simply adding overweight people to the existing categories of employees whose mere outward appearance prompts the kind of blind prejudice that leads to illegal labor practices.

Bottom Line

The foregoing is just a small sampling of the deluge of size discrimination currently occurring all over the United States. In 80 percent of the country—despite the Americans with Disabilities Act, the embryonic precedent of the Stouffer class-action suit, and the handful of other partial victories detailed above—the obese are fundamentally still on their own, prey to whatever punitive actions antifat employers care to dole out.

So, at least in the near future, the vast majority of pudgy plaintiffs are doomed to learn an expensive lesson: The social, psychological, and legal groundwork simply hasn't yet been laid for significant numbers of weight discrimination cases to prevail. Before that happens, antifat victims will have to wage the same sort of militant battles as did other oppressed groups, who marched in the streets to make it worthwhile to stride into the courtrooms.

7

Life With Laugh Track

....

Did you hear the one about the poor porker who got that horrible flesh-eating virus? Yeah, it's a real shame. They say she's only got ten years to live!

In a world where people agree on less and less as time goes by, there are two things we're unanimous about: Fat people are hilarious, and Fat Chicks are the most amusing of all. The only thing that's funnier still is a Fat Chick who actually thinks she's entitled to enjoy her life like a normal person. Laugh at this deluded loser and the world will laugh with you.

To a certain extent, this is just business as usual here on Planet Earth. The nature of the human beast seems to be that we always need a designated punching bag. So, if it's not a racial, ethnic, or religious minority, it's got to be some individual trait we can use to relegate somebody to lesser status than ourselves. Mercifully, most of us have finally evolved to a point where compassion has consigned such mindlessly cruel barbs to, if not extinction, at least a degree of odiousness that punishes anyone who still repeats them with a disapproving frown.

Some of us welcomed this overdue attitudinal transformation, which goes by the ambiguous name of "political correctness" (PC). Others had to be dragged to enlightenment, kicking and screaming about reverse discrimination every step of the way. And some are unrepentant still, though they've wised up enough to lower their voices and make sure they're among like-minded bigots before indulging in their nasty little knee-slappers.

But thanks to the billion-dollar brainwash, we've still got one allowable whipping girl left: our faithful, oh-so-useful friend, the Fat Chick. Stereotypically, she's sloppy, lazy, greedy, stupid, gross, clumsy, sweaty, smelly, antisocial, self-indulgent, hostile, loud, sarcastic, oversexed, and insensitive to the point of delusion. All of which means she's still fair game for any degree of cruelty anyone cares to inflict, especially if it's cloaked in the guise of humor. And the best part is, she won't fight back. She can't— there is no defense for all the negative qualities she represents.

So when she's a little girl, it's okay to trot out the timeworn "Fatty, fatty, two by four, couldn't get through the kitchen door." It's perfectly fine to make her sit red-cheeked and squirming through the many children's movies that include a stock fat-kid character who's not only always eating, but too dumb and food-obsessed to care what others think. *Little Giants*, say, or *Richie Rich*. Or *Casper*, in which the grossest of a trio of evil ghosts gobbles voraciously every moment it's on screen.

When the Fat Chick becomes a teenager, it's completely acceptable to hurl such "jests" as "Tubbo," "Lardo," "Porker," and "Blimpo" at her. If she doesn't like it, she can just stay home on prom night—when she certainly won't have a date anyway—and perhaps watch *Jurassic Park*, in which the chubby computer programmer played by Wayne Knight is a slob who constantly munches, speaks with his mouth full, strews his work area with food wrappers, and ends up betraying the good guys. Or Eddie Murphy's *The Nutty Professor*, which won the 1996 People's Choice Award despite containing an onslaught of gross, vulgar, stereotype-reinforcing fat jokes at the expense of its four-hundred-pound hero and his voracious family.

At school, amid the inevitable postprom giggling about the assorted weirdos who didn't show up, someone will make sure there's an audience to catch the Fat Chick's reaction to an old pop song that's carefully passed from generation to generation:

> I don't want her, you can have her
> She's too fat for me
> She's too fat, she's too fat
> She's too fat for me.

When the Fat Chick reaches adulthood, the jokey taunts can take on a whiff of sexual innuendo—"Thunder Thighs," "Bubble Butt," and the necessity of "pushin' through cushion"—just to make sure she doesn't miss the point about how far from ideal her body really is. "For a fat girl, you sure don't sweat much," she'll be told by way of flimsily veiled insult.

Other lessons regarding her status will be reiterated in nonstop comic quips during the course of any average day. When she's watching TV, for instance, she'll learn that

- being overweight automatically negates achievement. Not even prominent, successful, admired women can escape crude jokes about their figures. David Letterman, for example, has no qualms about cracking fat jokes about Oprah Winfrey—even since she's lost weight. (What kind of jokes? To pick just one in an outrageous onslaught: That Oprah's TV studio is plastered with zoolike signs saying "Please Don't Feed the Host.");
- comedian Joan Rivers, apparently forgetting she's on record as saying that "the psychic scars caused by believing you are ugly leave a permanent mark on your personality," will think nothing of claiming—among a flood of similar insults—that a photograph of Elizabeth Taylor on the cover of *People* "looks like she devoured her previous husbands."
- in nearly every episode of the otherwise charming *Home Improvement* series, the lead character, played by Tim Allen, cracks crude fat jokes at the expense of both his sidekick Al and Al's never-seen mother.

The lessons will continue even when the Fat Chick reads a book about losing weight:

- In *Diary of a Fat Housewife*, she'll note that author Rosemary Green takes Joan Rivers to task, albeit mildly, for joking about Elizabeth Taylor's weight, but only because she used Taylor's real name—implying that it's perfectly alright to ridicule fat people anonymously.

When the Fat Chick scans a newspaper, she'll see

• that students at The Citadel military academy in South Carolina were free to fight off female usurpers with purportedly humorous bumper stickers mocking wannabe-cadet Shannon Faulkner's famous extra twenty pounds: "Save the Males—Shave the Whale";

• that newspaper editors who need to round out a page with "filler" thank their lucky stars when something like this comes over the wire: "(AP) Seattle—A 410-pound death-row inmate is too fat to be hanged, a federal judge ruled . . . because he might be decapitated. . . .";

• or maybe it'll be a squib numerous news organizations found funny enough to print about an insensitive Florida teacher who got laughs by forcing an overweight student to wear a "Wide Load" sign. If the Fat Chick is lucky, this won't remind her of any humiliations in her own school days. (But if she's the author of this book, she'll remember a painful incident in the seventh grade when her gym teacher became angry because she had trouble learning to square-dance. She'll still see him stopping the music, rushing toward her, grabbing her and roughly shoving her through an intricate step. And when she kept on stumbling, how he stopped abruptly, stomped back up to the stage, and said to the entire class, "It's like trying to push a bull moose around.")

If the Fat Chick listens to a radio talk show, chances are good that she'll hear a typical exchange such as this:

NEWSCASTER: Did you hear the latest about Fergie?
D.J.: You mean the Duchess of *Pork*? What's she up to now?
NEWSCASTER: Seems she's gonna be Weight Watchers' newest shill.
D.J.: So does that mean she'll be talking about getting all that fat sucked out of the body—through her toes?!?

• Or "King of All Media" Howard Stern, who keeps even his most accomplished female guests in their place by fixating on how well they conform to his (and society's) notion of the ideal body, and who, while he may poke fun at everyone, seems to feel free to veer into outright cruelty when a woman is anything less than model-perfect;

• Or Michigan talk show host Ted Heusel inviting a representative of the National Association to Advance Fat Acceptance to talk about the fitness walk they've planned for International No-Diet Day (see Chapter 10), only to use his guest as the butt of simple-minded jokes. "So, are you gonna take an ambulance with you?"

Seeking a little comic relief, she'll find it hard to avoid cartoonists such as

• *B.C.*'s Johnny Hart, who created a horrendously aggressive character called "the fat broad" so he could make fun of her, decade after decade; or the venerable *Beetle Bailey* strip's Mort Walker, whose outrageously prejudicial jokes continue to victimize fat members of both sexes on a daily basis.

Browsing at the bookstore, she'll likely notice

• how much of the humor section is devoted to fat jokes. In a single book by Milton Berle (*Private Joke File*), there are no fewer than seventy. "She was so fat she went on her honeymoon in a U-Haul." "When she wears white she looks like a bandaged whale." "She never met a meal she didn't like."

Although it'll be small comfort, the Fat Chick will see that chunky men don't get off scot-free either:

• Watching an Academy Awards show, she'll wince when host David Letterman kicks off the evening with a tasteless, unfunny joke about portly film critic Roger Ebert devouring all of *Forrest Gump*'s notorious chocolates.
• Or she may be reminded of being fascinated as a child by the way Americans obviously loved to utter the full title of their leader: "the president of the United States of America," they'd say, always in respectful tones. But not today. Bill Clinton's weight has been average for his body type ever since he moved into the White House, and he jogs every morning, rain or shine.* But obesity is the ultimate leveler. So the myth that he's an out-of-control glutton has served as profitable fodder for comedians ranging from TV biggies like Leno, Letterman (again!), and the *Saturday Night Live* gang, right down to wee-hours deejays. And the print media are no bet-

*At least until a knee injury in 1997.

ter. In a typically gratuitous swipe, a recent fitness article in *Vogue* sarcastically denounced "the leader of the free world's double biceps curl—Quarter Pounder in one hand, slurpee in the other." Even when Clinton did lose a few pounds, *People* smirked: "Where's the blubba, bubba?"

• Venturing into a popular night spot, the Fat Chick may bump into the latest reincarnation of the bygone circus fat ladies: 300- and 400-pound sumo wrestlers with stage names such as Large Marge and Judy "The Bull" Jenkins, some of whom appear topless.

• And if she happens to be a journalist covering the inquest of a woman whose lifelong weight loss efforts killed her (see Chapter 11), she'll be horrified to hear the defendant's lawyer repeating a hoary old quip within earshot of the grieving family. "I'm not over-weight. I'm undertall!"

Laughing All the Way to the Bank

Whether or not we applaud the PC taboo against victimizing minori-ties, we have to notice that fat people are the only group that's still totally exempt from such social protection. If this contention strikes you as far-fetched, even in light of the foregoing examples, try substituting any racial, ethnic, or religious minority as the target of all these "jokes." Then ask yourself two questions: (1) Do the allegations implicit in each of the instances cited above—which include being ugly, unlovable, greedy, contemptible, gluttonous, cannibalistic, bestial, feeble, belliger-ent, and self-deceiving—still seem like harmless fun? And (2) Would such assertions be socially tolerated in any other context?

The universal contempt that preserves Fat Chicks' status as society's last allowable laughing stock didn't just happen. Certainly many indi-viduals, both famous and private, revel in ridiculing the obese for fun and profit. But the lion's share of the blame for deliberately escalating and perpetuating antifat bigotry undeniably goes to the weight loss profiteers. They saw that there was a fortune to be made by exploit-ing one of the baser human inclinations, which is enhancing self-esteem by denigrating "inferiors." Or, as novelist Daniel Pinkwater describes this: "There is nothing we humans like better than abusing and reviling others for perceived faults of which we are guilty our-selves—but are getting away with."

Thus, the strategy of turning up the cultural heat on Fat Chicks coerces them into spending every penny they possibly can to try to escape the orchestrated punishment. And the vivid object lessons, in turn, pressure smaller women into spending whatever it takes to avoid being included in the vilified group.

Meanwhile, the remainder of the population also absorbs antifat messages and responds to Pavlovian reinforcement right on cue by mocking the obese at every opportunity. Media wordsmiths get in on the fun by concocting sneering phrases such as "gravitationally chal-lenged," "horizontally challenged," "human heftiness," "diametrically disadvantaged," and "St. Oprah of the Stairmaster." Finally, the mind-less monkey-see-monkey-do tradition is passed on to children. Result: Everlasting profits are guaranteed to roll in.

But exactly which mental buttons are being pushed when someone jeers at a Fat Chick and someone else laughs? Mark Breslin believes a couple of them serve the billion-dollar brainwash perfectly. As founder of the national Yuk Yuk's Comedy Club chain, he says he's noticed that a lot of humor springs from "fear that our body will betray us at any minute by spiraling out of control—whether it's through sex or size." Breslin also believes that ambivalence about breaking rules is another of our psychological buttons. He's been watching audiences for a long time now and knows the exhilaration people feel when societal con-ventions are flagrantly flouted. "But it all depends on who's doing it," he told me. "Some people can get away with it and some can't."

One who can't, at least in the view of her legions of irate critics, is comic actress Roseanne (formerly surnamed Barr and Arnold) because she pushes both of these mental buttons, according to Breslin. "She's just too much for most people to take. She's overweight, has a big mouth, and presents herself as working class. Yet she earns a gazillion dollars and enjoys all the rewards that are 'supposed' to go to svelte, conventionally attractive women."

Comedian Kathi Maio couldn't agree more. And she believes that what also makes Roseanne a target for intense anger is that she broke a crucial silence. As Maio writes in *Revolutionary Laughter: The*

World of Women Comics, before Roseanne "entered our living rooms
. . . like an invading army of Amazons . . . women of substance led a
shamefaced, completely secondary existence in our culture. . . . [She]
exposed the female experience by exposing herself. . . . And she made
it clear that she wasn't going to put up with any bullshit about her
jeans size."

Bingo! To people who've been carefully brainwashed to believe that
Fat Chicks should sit down, shut up, and have the decency to be
ashamed of themselves, Roseanne's exuberant defiance is so bewildering it makes the arrows on their mental compasses gyrate wildly. If she's
allowed to get away with that attitude, nothing in their lives will make
sense anymore. There'll simply be no way of knowing which way is up.

Now try another swap. Insert into the bumpy scenario of Roseanne's
career the name of anyone who personifies an excluded minority. Then
ask yourself if the venomous response to Roseanne's refusal to accept
her assigned role (i.e., shamefaced Fat Chick) isn't identical to the
mental process that produces every other kind of prejudice. If "these
people" aren't put in "their place," p.d.q., some of us are afraid our little world will wobble so violently we won't know who's who anymore.
Or, more to the point, whether *we* are still happily occupying the high
hierarchical rank we desire—and have convinced ourselves we
deserve. Far better to take no chances, and nail everything down with
a clear understanding of the rules, an agreement among ourselves to
abide by them, and severe penalties for anyone who disobeys.

But how can we disseminate and enforce these vital rules? Simple.
Just ape the technique of demagogues since time immemorial, be they
ambitious dictators, unscrupulous politicians, callous royals, religious
fanatics, or marketing moguls. First, decide what you want and who
you're most likely to swindle it from. Then designate that group as an
"enemy of the people" and shout it from the rooftops. If you demonize and dehumanize your target convincingly enough, rather than
being outraged, everyone else will be so relieved they're not among
the outcasts that they'll do everything in their power to maintain the
status quo. After which you won't have to lift a finger—except, of
course, to count your profits. Thy will will be done until earth becomes
heaven for you and hell for your victims.

Makes sense. But isn't "demonize and dehumanize" a tad strong? Not at all. Let's take the most obvious example of all: war. History is drenched with bloody examples. Somebody covets somebody else's land, or gold, or oil, or widgets. So the first somebody hauls out the biggest saber available and starts rattling it passionately. That so-and-so has no right to those widgets! He/she/it is nothing but a useless, worthless, disgusting blankety-blank.

And everybody knows blankety-blanks eat their young, despoil our precious world, and slither on their bellies like reptiles! A reptile doesn't deserve widgets, now does it? We deserve them because we embody everything the blankety-blanks do not. We're clean, upstanding, hard working, virtuous, brave, and, above all, human. Which means not only that we are vastly superior to the dastardly blankety-blanks, but that the Almighty is automatically on our side—and wants us to show those wicked, serpentine, Almighty-less blankety-blanks who's who. We must strive to deserve the Almighty's favor by doing the Almighty's will—which is to trounce the blankety-blanks once and for all and take the widgets that are rightfully ours. And that means war, my friends. Forward, ho!

Fattening 'Em Up for the Kill

Now let's fill in the blankety-blanks and see how well humor acts as one more big gun in the arsenal of weapons the pillaging propagandists use to swipe the Fat Chicks' treasure and that of her slimmer sisters. Let's start by deconstructing a few antiobesity gags:

• A fat, well-dressed, ultra-dignified woman is strolling down a boulevard when she notices a bedraggled, extremely inebriated man staring at her and chuckling. "Lady," says the drunk, "you are the fattest person I've ever seen." "And you," she replies in her snootiest tone, "are the drunkest person I've ever seen." "Yeah," the wino replies, "but I'll be sober in the morning."
• A sleazy strip joint in the Midwest carves out a cachet for itself by advertising "50 Beautiful Girls and 3 Ugly Ones." How ugly are we talking? Well, to be honest, the only strippers who answered the ads weren't all that bad-looking. But some of them are pudgy, so

management is home free. The joint is guaranteed to go hog wild when these gals doff their duds and let it *all* hang out!

• A neophyte comic climbs on stage at a club whose clientele is accustomed to more seasoned acts. It looks like disaster time when his ho-hum schtick bombs and a heckler down front revs up his harassment. Then the comic spies an escape route. He'll just aim his half-baked barbs straight at the heckler and keep tacking on "ya fat pig." It works. His jibes bring the house down, and everyone goes home happy.

What's really going on here? And how do such scenarios fatten the antifat profiteers' bottom lines? By using what virtually amounts to a new form of Esperanto in which accusing someone of being obese is understood to be the equivalent of exposing their dirty little secret and shattering their "pretense" of respectability.

It's the same kind of detestable mind game that used to be considered acceptable in the context of racial, ethnic, and religious minorities. Belly laughs could always be won by simply imitating, or alluding to, gross stereotypes. And gutter epithets acted as code that instantly communicated a reprehensible subtext: It's okay to laugh because the blankety-blanks aren't like "us." They're a lesser species. They must be, or everyone wouldn't be laughing so hard. By inference, this makes everyone who doesn't belong to the target *du jour* superior—no matter how much evidence there is to the contrary. Even if we're hopeless drunkards, pot-bellied strip-club patrons with nowhere better to go, or dullard descendants of the bear baiters of yore hanging around clubs to heckle the comedians. Hey, at least we're not despicable blankety-blanks. So all's right with the world.

F—the Last Scarlet Letter

A halt to this kind of cruel, divisive, culture-coarsening bigot humor has been called by the PC movement. But the sole remaining variation on the theme—that Fat Chicks are the worst blankety-blanks of all—remains intact thanks to three decades of incessant antifat propaganda. Consequently, any transgressor who dares to buck "conventional wisdom" is rocking the profit boat and must pay a heavy price.

Roseanne is at the top of the list of Fat Chicks whose refusal to be cowed threatens the aggressively entrenched scheme of things. The worst venom was sprayed after Roseanne's parody of ballpark anthem singers went awry a few years ago. But vituperation also reached a fever pitch after her appearances on the cover of *Vanity Fair* magazine, wearing scanty lingerie and an unmistakably in-your-face expression. Displaying such a large body so shamelessly was regarded as tantamount to committing a crime. Theft, most likely, because everyone knows the covers of popular magazines are reserved for women who have the decency to do what they're told, which is whittle their bodies down to skin and bones, complemented by big, surgically augmented breasts.

Second case in point: Oprah Winfrey. As a two-fer who was both fat and from a minority, she simply had no business being so talented and hardworking that she's predicted to become the first African-American billionaire in U.S. history. So pundits crowed when she first lost weight and then began regaining it, while the tabloids chronicled every pound: "Oprah passes 200!" But slimming down again only compounded her perceived impertinence—infuriating, rather than placating, the antifat forces. Why? Because if Fat Chicks achieve mega-success, theories about their inferiority will fly out the window and the whole hoax may be exposed.

Does Winfrey feel she's been punished accordingly? Definitely. She kicked off a show in early 1994 gazing at a TV monitor as videotape rolled from several of the series that have lampooned her the most mercilessly: *In Living Color, Seinfeld, Saturday Night Live*, and, of course, *Late Show With David Letterman*. And this is to say nothing of the thousands of jokes still told around the continent about her formerly rotund figure.

Fun 'n' Games on the Flip Side

Until these admirable women* achieved monumental success—on their own terms—Fat Chicks who could successfully fend off the orchestrated onslaught of bigot humor were few and far between. But

*And Rosie O'Donnell, whose stereotype-smashing career is disussed in Chapter 12.

here comes the good news: The tide is now turning big-time (double entendre purely intentional). Other facets of what's gradually becoming an exciting fight-back revolution, reminiscent of women's liberation and the civil rights movement, are detailed in Chapter 10. But I've clustered some of the most humorous of the ongoing efforts here as a bracing antidote to the heartless "comedy" described above.

Welcoming Back Womanly Sized Women: Plump playwright Wendy Wasserstein, whose highly regarded Broadway productions include *The Heidi Chronicles*, somehow managed to mesmerize *Harper's Bazaar* into printing a fable that contradicted pretty much everything the posh magazine stands for. Actually, her piece was probably intended as damage control for Tina Gaudoin's detestable denial a few months earlier that portraying only ultra-thin models encourages eating disorders.

Wasserstein's fantasy was titled "Goodbye Waif, Hello Bulge." The heroine of the hilarious what-if story is a Junoesque, 183-pound model named Wanderful who transforms the fashion scene after being discovered in a Kansas City diner while wolfing down biscuits and gravy. Before long, "hips and thighs return to American couture in a big way," and formerly successful supermodels like Cindy Crawford steal away "to fat farms, where they binge on cholesterol." Meanwhile, the fashionable new "bulge look makes thin women feel [so] embarrassed about their flat tummies . . . that they [begin] gorging themselves on Heath Bar Crunch ice cream and duck sausage [and] avoiding exercise." Wasserstein's welcome parody ends with a goofy but pointed refutation of Gaudoin's own words: "Eating disorders don't come from fashion. They are a dysfunction of dysfunction . . . [and] the fact that thin women are unable to be happy with their well-toned bodies has nothing to do with the current bulge trend."

Waving Goodbye to the Waifs: Jay Leno's audience cracked up one night in the spring of 1995 when a female guest told what may well be the world's first bona fide antibulimia joke. It concerned something that sounds like, but is not, a gag in itself: Several of the skinniest supermodels (Elle MacPherson, Naomi Campbell, Claudia Schiffer, and Christy Turlington) recently opened a restaurant at New York's famed Rockefeller Center. Logically enough, it's called the Fashion Cafe.

Here's the joke: "A customer comes in, sits down, and orders a lima bean shake. It's so nauseating that she calls the waiter over and says: 'I feel like I'm going to throw up.' And the waiter replies: 'Exactly!' "

Crimes of Corpulence: When she was still Rubenesque, Kathy Najimy,* who was so appealing as the relentlessly upbeat nun in the two *Sister Act* movies that she was tapped to star in the opening dance number at the 1995 Academy Awards, and included as one of *In Style* magazine's "heavenly bodies," tipped off late-night TV talk host Greg Kinnear about Los Angeles's antifat laws: "If you're five pounds overweight, you only have to pay a five-dollar ticket. Being fifteen pounds overweight gets you a fifteen-dollar misdemeanor ticket. But twenty pounds is a felony. And fifty pounds automatically means the electric chair."

Mind Over Matter: Writer Mickey Guisewite turns out to be just as amusingly perspicacious as her cartoonist sister, Cathy. The duo recently collaborated on a book of comic essays titled *Dancing Through Life in a Pair of Broken High Heels.* Arguably the best chapter is "I Think, Therefore I am Fat," which begins: "The reason men will never understand women's weight anxiety is because men have never had to get on the same scale we do: The one that is in our brains. The one that tells us every morning that we're fat. The one that reminds us all day long that we're fat. . . . The one that makes us overeat because, what the heck, we're already fat."

Destruction by Deconstruction: For the past five years, a unique troupe of Vancouver "culture jammers," called the Media Foundation, has used caustically humorous "subvertising" to help readers of its *Adbusters* magazine become "media literate" enough to perceive the ghastly underside of many of the most ubiquitous ad campaigns. Logically enough, much of their efforts concern the work of antifat profiteers. A favorite target is Calvin Klein, whose advertising for Obsession perfume the group has metamorphosed into a soft-focus, black and white photo of a woman's nude torso. "Obsessed" reads the headline,

*Najimy has since slimmed down.

with the credit line going to "Calvin Swine." On second glance, you realize that the ad brings bulimia right out in the open, because the woman is crouched over a toilet. The Media Foundation shot a television version of this hard-hitting, advertiser-offending spot two years ago and has been pitching it to networks ever since. But so far, none has allowed the radical group to buy time to air the spot.

Bottom Line

Antifat humor is *not* harmless fun; it is the sole surviving form of socially acceptable discrimination. And to complain about it is not simply to throw a "pity party" for Fat Chicks. For what's so destructive about this brand of bigot comedy isn't just that it hurts the feelings and restricts the lives of large females, young, older, and yet to be born. It also undermines tolerance for diversity throughout our society, helping to keep us divided into sparring factions. And nothing could be more useful to the imagemeisters than this classic divide-and-conquer technique.

The welcome "reverse humor" trend promises to be a very effective revolutionary tool over time. It also seems like such good, therapeutic fun that I can't resist trying my own hand at it.

THE SCENE: Some late night in the sweet by-and-by in beautiful downtown wherever, at the popular If The Tables Were Turned comedy club. On stage is a jolly jokester who's just winding up the last set of the evening. Let's listen:

But seriously, ladies and germs, you've been a great audience—for skinny folks! Yeah, I know what your problem is. You're afraid your scrawny little bones'll shatter if you crack up, right? And who's got enough energy to applaud when all you're eating is a couple of lettuce leaves and half an eye of newt—hold the dressing? And that's only on days starting with a W!

Ba-boom.

Anyhoo, let's wrap it up tonight with a really cheap shot. How cheap is it? It's sooooo cheap you can afford it even after you've paid your dues at Jenny Watchers, or wherever the hell you go to make sure your ego doesn't get too healthy. It's sooooo tasteless that even those yucky diet-food makers won't use it as an ingredient. Ready? Here goes.

Two gals walk into a restroom. They take one look at their bony little bods in the mirror, shake their heads in dismay, head into the stalls, and stick their fingers down their throats. Between heaves, one manages to gasp: "You know what I can't believe?" "What?" croaks the other. "That only one diet doctor has been shot to death so far!"

Ba-boom.

8

Starved for Affection

....

Her suitor was amorous and persistent. He had proposed marriage over and over again, but she always turned him down because she cherished her independence and her stage career, to say nothing of her international reputation as the most desirable woman of the 1890s.

Today, however, the big man with the huge gem in his cravat was determined to hear "yes." He strode into her salon, took one look at her cornflower blue eyes, peaches-and-cream complexion, and the two hundred pounds of dimpled flesh flowing into a perfect hourglass, and decided to play his trump card.

"Sit down, darling," said Diamond Jim Brady to Lillian Russell. And when she did, he poured a million dollars into her capacious lap.

Her answer to his proposal was still no. But that didn't end their liaison, and they continued doing all the things they enjoyed most. Eating together was so high on the list of their favorite pastimes that Russell once won a diamond ring Brady offered her if she could consume as much as he did.

Luscious Lillian wouldn't fare quite so well a century later. Instead of being celebrated as "sonnets of motion," her ample curves would be so despised and denigrated by others that she'd probably detest the sight of them herself. Her chances of meeting, let alone attracting the love of, a top tycoon would be zilch. Star status and international admiration would be out of the question. And if she allowed herself to gorge on her favorite foods, it certainly wouldn't be in the company of a man whose esteem she valued. Anyway, she'd probably either force herself to regurgitate her feast or loathe and berate herself for eating it in the first place.

All in all, if Lillian Russell were somehow transported to the 1990s, her first response to the new world would probably be utter incredulity. Since the beginning of time, her explicitly fertile body type has been favored by nature, men, and artists. But today she'd be told in no uncertain terms, and by any number of sources, that she represented the epitome of ugliness—simply because her weight was almost twice what's now allowable for any woman who wishes to be considered attractive.

In our day, Lillian would have to look long and hard to find any successful, celebrated, or abundantly beloved women whose girth remotely resembled hers. Flipping through magazines or newspapers wouldn't do it. And if she figured out how to turn on a TV set, she'd likely recoil in horror at the sight of the skeletal, near-naked young women who slither and grind through music videos. Then she'd channel-surf until her thumb got sore, looking for large ladies. Zap: Skinny women and girls fretting about their shameful appetites. Zap: Skinny women in peril after abusive peril. Zap: A skinny blonde excitedly flipping alphabet letters. Zap: Skinny yet strangely busty women prancing in bathing suits. Zap: Skinny women reporting the news. Zap, zap, zap: More of the same.

With luck, though, Lillian might stumble upon a performance by Aretha Franklin or Wynonna, the only large female superstars left in North American music. Although Lil wouldn't know it, there used to be others: Kate Smith, Mahalia Jackson, Sophie Tucker, Mama Cass. But not now.

Zapping onward, Lillian might catch irrepressible Rosie O'Donnell's talk show. Or large-and-lovely Liz Torres on *The John Laroquette Show*. Or ample Elaine Miles on *Northern Exposure*. Or curvy Isabel Sanford on *The Jeffersons*. Or stout Conchata Ferrell on *Hearts Afire*. Or portly Kathy Kinney on *The Drew Carey Show*. Or Junoesque Camryn Manheim playing an opinionated lawyer, Eleanor, on *The Practice*.

But, as something of an expert on romance, Lillian would surely notice that these substantial women rarely get to play love scenes. In fact, when a character Ferrell portrayed in a different TV series—*L.A. Law*—married an extremely handsome man, the other characters expressed incredulity because of her size. Sure enough, one plot twist later, it turned out that the marriage was just a sham to get the man a "green card" that allowed him to remain in the United States.

If her timing was right, however, Lillian would discover *Roseanne*, the only series in the history of television starring (and created by) a Fat Chick whose weight doesn't relegate her to the status of self-deprecating buffoon or pitiful spinster or both. The show is also unique in that it depicts a married couple* who were both hefty but whose size was incidental to the plot lines, and whose love and sexual attraction for each other were unmistakable.

Alternatively, Lillian might catch *Avonlea*, in which Lally Cadeau (who plays Janet King), while certainly not a two-hundred-pounder, does resemble the well-rounded women of her character's Edwardian era and enjoys an obviously amorous relationship with her screen husband.

But if Lillian became encouraged enough by these few shows to assume she'd find similar dynamics in any other media images today, she'd be disappointed. And bewildered—because on the street, in stores and offices, on public transportation, and everywhere else, she'd see more real women who do look like her than scrawny waifs who do not.

"What in tarnation," she might well ask us, "have you done to yourselves in a hundred years?"

What we've done is surrendered even such a fundamental of human life as love to the forces of commercialization. Beauty is still in the eye of the beholder, just as it was a century ago. But the minds that see through those eyes have been brainwashed to condemn and exclude every physical quality that doesn't serve the interests of marketers. In the 1990s, even though we believe we're the freest thinkers in history, our psyches and libidos are virtually owned by the big-bucks industries of diet, fitness, fashion, beauty, and cosmetic surgery.

*At least until Roseanne and Dan's separation during the 1996–97 TV season.

So, above all, men must not find heavy women desirable, because that might stop all women from spending billions of dollars on whatever promises corporeal salvation. Above all, women must not consider themselves attractive unless they're clones of the emaciated, painted, surgically and photographically enhanced beauty icons who now dominate all forms of popular culture.

That leaves rather a lot of us out in the cold.

For the record, there *are* some large women who are happily attached. They and their significant others are to be congratulated for staying sane while the rest of us succumbed to the billion-dollar brainwash.

And succumb we did, body and soul. Three decades into the No Fat Chicks era, the vast majority of adults, teenagers, and children now believe that large women are disgusting, unforgivable, and—in the context of romance—a caste of untouchables.

Does that statement strike you as exaggerated? Then consider a recent survey of male college students concerning what type of woman they'd be least likely to marry. Fat Chicks "won," ranking as less appealing than cocaine users, shoplifters, embezzlers, and ex–mental patients.

Or you could check out the personals ads in your local newspaper and count how many male romance-seekers specify slim, thin, fit, or variations on the theme. More than 80 percent of the personals ads in a recent edition of the Louisville, Kentucky, *Courier-Journal*, for instance, included such demands. There was also one that simply thundered: "No fatties."

According to a recent study by the Harvard School of Public Health, large women are at least 20 percent less likely to marry than their thinner counterparts. Divorce and marital discord are also disproportionately prevalent for fat women, according to a welter of anecdotal evidence (although no scientific studies appear to have been done).

Advice columns frequently feature letters similar to a recent one to Ann Landers from an Arizona man who complained that he'd been "forced into celibacy" for the past ten years because his wife had gained weight. Another man was convicted in Tennessee of attempting to have his wife killed (on Mother's Day!) because she hadn't lost the weight she put on during pregnancy.

Two men who appeared on the *Carnie* TV talk show—entitled "They Hate Me Just Because I'm Fat"—stopped short of murder, but bald-facedly maligned their romantic partners for gaining weight. The first grouched that "she's done the most unforgivable thing a woman can do to her man." But when his wife strolled onto the set wearing shorts, she appeared to weigh no more than 130 pounds. The other man, insisting that his fiancée was "a beautiful person" but that he just couldn't "deal with the fat," had recently invited her to lunch, but taken her instead to a fitness center, where he'd secretly signed her up for membership. The tall woman in question looked to be a statuesque 160 at most.

Granted, those are extreme examples of fat-phobia. But it's equally sad and wasteful when so many other heavy women endure lifetimes of romantic exclusion—from not receiving valentine cards in grade school, to missing proms in high school, to being wallflowers at college mixers, to being ignored or insulted in singles spots as adults. And, of course, this kind of ostracism is often in addition to being left out of the kind of everyday social life that affords opportunities to meet potential mates.

Small wonder that, as Roberta Pollack Seid remarks in *Never Too Thin: Why Women Are at War With Their Bodies*, "many women regard their weight as the central issue of their lives, the primary obstacle to self-realization, the matter that must be resolved before other issues, such as careers or romance, can be addressed."

The Fat Lady Vanishes

Overweight women are punished and penalized for their appearance in many facets of their lives. But as tough as it is to lose out in economic, social, and practical matters, being disqualified from romantic relationships can be even more devastating. "Because 'beauty' lives so deep in the psyche, where sexuality mingles with self-esteem," Naomi Wolf explains in *The Beauty Myth*, "to tell a woman she is ugly can make her feel ugly, act ugly, and . . . be ugly, in the place where feeling beautiful keeps her whole."

Put another way, as Whitney Otto writes in *Now You See Her*: "The inside soon listens to the outside and the next thing you know, you're a ghost." This perceptive novel actually chronicles what often happens as women age (another branch of the billion-dollar brainwash). But Fat Chicks frequently respond in the same self-defeating way to the inescapable message that they are undesirable and unwanted. That is, they retreat into the "ghosthood" of protective isolation and living only "from the neck up."

So, if no man can get anywhere near them, they eliminate the risk of being rejected. If they never go near "date bait" bars and restaurants, they won't be subjected to cruel critiques of their appearance— or, even worse, crude jokes about the sexual insatiability of women who appear to have large appetites.

Whatever situation they happen to be in, they're extremely careful to avoid the appearance of flirting, lest it provide fodder for yet another cruel jest. This motivation can extend as far as actually reassuring any man they're talking to—using a variety of verbal and non-verbal techniques—that they know there's no possibility he will find her sexually attractive. In this context, I remember my closest friend scolding me that, when we were at social gatherings, she would usually see me erecting an invisible, man-repelling barrier of defensiveness around myself as if to say: Don't even think about approaching me because I know, and you know, that nothing will come of it.

In an attempt to avoid painful misunderstandings in such situations, Fat Chicks often spin out whole social scenarios in their heads of how a romantic catastrophe might occur. They write all the dialogue, control all the imaginary action, and inevitably cast themselves as losers. Logically enough, this can lead to habitual isolation. Such protective reclusiveness can, in turn, become a self-perpetuating trap that makes any kind of social contact—romantic or otherwise—more and more intimidating as time goes by. In extreme cases, such isolation can turn into a condition closely resembling an agoraphobic's panic about leaving home.

But at least that's not as self-destructive, or physically dangerous, as the degrading promiscuity to which desperate loneliness sometimes drives overweight women. And too many of the men they attract are on the lookout for women whose frail self-esteem makes them highly exploitable. A particularly appalling example of this dynamic recently occurred in Toronto when a physician lost his medical license for, among other offenses against his obese female patients, coercing a woman into having sex in return for getting her stomach stapled.

Other large women find different ways to hide. "When I was thin, I couldn't say no to my husband if he wanted sex. If I looked gorgeous—which meant thin—I assumed my body belonged to him," a woman named Lisa told the authors of *When Women Stop Hating Their Bodies*. "Somehow when I'm fat," she continued, "I'm not Daddy's little girl in the same way. [So] I worry that if I lose weight, I'll lose myself again."

The I-Deserve-It Syndrome

For heavy women who've been too demoralized to defend themselves any other way, being alone affords plenty of time to come up with corroboration—and therefore psychological justification—for the prejudice that envelops them. Put another way, if they can find a way to blame *themselves*, the pain and prejudice will make some kind of sense and be infinitesimally easier to bear.

Which sometimes leads Fat Chicks to think such thoughts as these: "I happened to glance down at my body," wrote Margaret Atwood in an illuminating novel, *Lady Oracle*, "[and] there, staring me in the face, was my thigh. It was enormous, it was gross, it was like a diseased limb . . . it spread on forever, like a prairie photographed from a plane . . . with veins meandering across it like rivers. It was the size of three ordinary thighs."

The operative word in Atwood's insightful passage is, of course, "ordinary." For large women have been just as brainwashed as everyone else into denigrating any manifestation of "ordinary" or "normal" that doesn't match the media's standard. And if you're so convinced your body is disgusting that even appearing fully clothed is an ordeal, the prospect of revealing your naked body—even for lovemaking—can seem like an utter impossibility.

So even if a Fat Chick *is* in a relationship, the shame she's internalized can poison the couple's sex life. A brave woman named Michelle Hrabak, for example, recently told *Ladies' Home Journal* that, when she weighed 257 pounds, her husband "still wanted to make love, but I could barely get undressed in front of him, let alone deal with having him touch my hip bulges. Then, I'd only make love with the lights out. . . . Finally, I just shut down—wasn't interested in sex at all."

Similar body anxiety is expressed in an intriguing article about posing for a photo exhibition "exploring the erotic possibilities of an unconventional body" in a recent issue of *Extra!* San Francisco writer Laura Fraser, who participated in the exhibition, points out that "many of us have spent more time in bed pulling our stomachs in than letting our passions loose." If that sounds preposterous, let me remind you that, not so long ago, *Cosmopolitan* published an article with detailed instructions about the best ways for women to pose and position themselves during lovemaking so they won't look fat!

Many of the women who responded to my Internet bulletin and *USA Today* ad expressed crushing sexual inhibition because of their appearance. This was scarcely a surprise, since numerous surveys show that, no matter what they weigh, as many as 90 percent of women feel bad about their bodies. That leaves only a tiny minority whose sense of attractiveness hasn't been so undermined that their sexual confidence is in tatters.

The authors of *Feminist Perspectives on Eating Disorders* vividly describe this kind of psychological damage: "The tyranny of the ideal image makes almost all of us feel inferior. An internal voice rages at us: 'You are fat. You are ugly. Your thighs are like jelly. You have cellulite. You have pimples. You have vaginal odor. Your hair is drab. Your skin is dry.' We are taught to hate our bodies, and thus learn to hate ourselves."

He's Ashamed to Be Seen With Me and Other Sad Tales

Several of my respondents reported that their partners are ashamed to be seen with them in public or among male friends or professional colleagues. And I, too, remembered "only-in-the-dark dating," as a woman from New York termed it, and especially a boyfriend with whom I lived for several years who—on the rare occasions when he didn't succeed in keeping his acquaintances from meeting me—habitually introduced me as his "tenant."

Some women described how they passively put up with various degrees of abuse for fear of losing their husbands or lovers and then not being able to attract anyone else. And more than one said her husband had admitted feeling shortchanged because his partner didn't measure up to the "trophy woman" image he's been conditioned to feel he deserves.

Darla, from Chicago, wrote about how devastated she felt the first time she made love with a man she'd yearned for for years, only to hear him say, "as if he never noticed till then, that I was 'a really big girl.'" Caroline, from Seattle, described the lengths to which she goes to avoid letting men she's interested in see her from the rear. "Even if it's time for me to go home, or if I urgently need to go to the bathroom, if I can't get out without keeping my back to the wall, I just sit there."

Carol, from Atlanta, said that "there are only about two days a year when I don't hate my looks so much I'm afraid to set foot out my door." Sandy, from Austin, said that whenever she tried to visualize herself "getting intimate with someone, my fantasy would be shattered because I knew I couldn't find lingerie that would make me look even halfway like I should."

And a correspondent from Toronto, who identified herself only as "Wasted," cracked a bitter joke about being "a double virgin now, because every cell in the body is renewed over seven years, and it's been fourteen years since I've had sex."

He Must Be Crazy If He Thinks I'm Attractive

Doing an attitudinal about-face when someone actually admires the body that everyone else despises is very difficult, according to some of my other respondents, who reported being unable to accept or trust men who do appreciate their ample appearance. These comments reminded me of a time when I was a young legal secretary. There was a client who was so crazy about my chunky legs that, every time he had an appointment with my boss, he'd arrive, say, "Hi, Terry," stare at my legs, and walk right into the wall. Any other woman would probably have been flattered. But all I remember thinking was, "What's wrong with this weirdo?"

A large woman in an extraordinary documentary film called *Fat Chance* (discussed in Chapter 12) goes much farther in this same vein: "I've been told so many times that I have 'such a beautiful face' that now, when I hear it, I want to mutilate myself so people will stop saying it." As sad as this statement is, it nevertheless demonstrates that the woman has not bought into the ugly-duckling-becomes-gorgeous-swan fairy tale that's implicit in the nonstop makeover features that permeate women's magazines. (Sample headline: "My Husband Fell in Love With a 'New' Woman, and It Was Me!")

Marcia Millman explains the entrapping effect of the before-and-after fantasy in a moving book called *Such a Pretty Face: Being Fat in America*: "The need to be extraordinarily beautiful is related to the need for unconditional love. So severe was the original rejection and injury, that it is not enough to be average."

The internal and external obsession with women's appearance, which is deliberately instilled by the weight-loss and beauty industries, is reflected in all of these comments. Which brings to mind Anaïs Nin's famous axiom: "We don't see things as they are, we see them as we are."

Many of the conflicted feelings expressed by my respondents also shine a big spotlight on a 1989 survey by *Vogue* magazine in which a majority of the women participants stated that, in return for having "ideal figures," they would willingly give up their husbands and boyfriends (as well as their careers and money). This defeat-the-purpose attitude shows just how far from human verities we all have been dragged. The age-old practice of trying to attract a mate by looking beautiful has been co-opted into a pathetically self-contained, self-focused effort that has lonely, exhausted, obsessed women running in place and getting nowhere—except to the gym and the mall.

What About Men?

Men who've absorbed the No Fat Chicks credo are all too numerous, not to mention all too vociferous on occasion. Of course, having attractive women on their arms has been a status symbol for men for hundreds of years. But if there are any Diamond Jim Bradys left in North America today, they're keeping mighty quiet. In fact, the very thought of a Donald Trump becoming besotted with a woman the size of, say, Roseanne seems even less likely than the notion that the controversial multimillionaire might toss all his money from the top of one of his skyscrapers.

But there *are* some men who've managed to resist the brainwashing and are attracted to large women despite—or because of—their size. The bravest of these guys say so right out loud. And a few lionhearts actually do so in front of their buddies, knowing that the resulting flak, raucous remarks, and innuendo about their masculinity are bound to be brutal.

A couple of these independent thinkers have even written books about their love for plus-size women. In *Fat Is Not a Four-Letter Word*, for instance, physiologist Charles Roy Schroeder states that his wife, whom "most people in our culture would consider to be fat," was wearing a bathing suit the first time they met. "And before I ever said a word to her," Schroeder recalls, "my hormones started bubbling."

One of William Fabrey's motivations for helping found the National Association to Advance Fat Acceptance was that, while applying for their marriage license, his plus-size wife-to-be was asked by a clerk who could possibly be interested in marrying her.

Fashion photographer Ken Mayer is another bold soul who has backed up his beliefs in a book and in many media appearances, including a memorable *Donahue* show during which he spiritedly defended his fellow "fat-admirers"—many of whom, he said, remain "in the closet because society discriminates against them." In *Real Women Don't Diet: One Man's Praise of Large Women and His Outrage at the Society That Rejects Them*, Mayer muses, "I think I'm a throwback to what men are all about." He also gets deliciously truculent (from a Fat Chick's point of view, that is) in his denunciation of a culture that "worship[s] the too-thin, childlike female body [and] limits their happiness at every turn."

As we'll see in Chapter 10, large women and the men who find them attractive have recently begun coming up with creative ways of finding each other. But, even though Schroeder's and Mayer's praise is music to a Fat Chick's ears, such men don't have an easy time breaking down the defenses of women who've been scarred for life by antifat prejudice.

Dan Davis, an accountant whose views resemble those of Mayer and Schroeder, recently focused on this stumbling block in a revealing article in *Radiance* magazine: "Fat women are often harder to approach than thin women. Because of the psychological battering inflicted on them by society, many ... become defensive and withdrawn. Suspicious of compliments, they may be annoyed or baffled by even the sincerest admirer [whereas] thin women are much more likely to accept male attention as their due."

And How About Children?

There may be no sadder result of the billion-dollar brainwash than the fact that, if heavy women have fewer marriages and romantic relationships than their slimmer sisters, they're also less likely to have children. Actual statistics, however, proved impossible to elicit. In fact, many of those to whom I put my queries either couldn't fathom what I was getting at or responded in such sarcastic tones that they may just as well have come out and said what they obviously were thinking: "Who cares about fat women anyway?"

Compounding the cruel social attitudes that prevent Fat Chicks from bearing their own children is the fact that obesity is viewed so negatively by many adoption authorities—who spout the same fallacious health issues as do the employers discussed in Chapter 6—that extra pounds are frequently considered an automatic disqualifier.

Bottom Line

Zaftig Kathy Bates was asked in a recent interview how it felt to be passed over in favor of slimmer actresses for the movie versions of several roles she triumphantly created on stage. The thoughtful answer given by the multi-award-winning Bates extended well beyond her own self-interest: "We've been taught to accept this very narrow definition of what is beautiful for women, and we are missing the humanity in people because of what someone may happen to look like."

Her eloquent remark resonates powerfully in the context of romantic love, as it is experienced by—and withheld from—large women, in the destructive wake of social conditioning since the exploitation of

Twiggymania. Throughout most of recorded history, Rubenesque damsels were deemed the ideal "squeeze." But today, when even the most intimate relationships between human beings have been commodified and manipulated accordingly by media images, millions of women who resemble the celebrated Lillian Russell lead lonely, loveless, conflicted lives and are often bereft of husbands, children, and grandchildren.

The profitable plundering of psyches has affected both sides of the romantic equation. Yet most of the men who feel repelled by Fat Chicks are merely behaving as they've been deliberately trained to do over the past three decades. And many large women, who've been equally hoodwinked, are blind to both their own innate worth and to the admirers with whom they might find fulfilling relationships. Geneen Roth explains the sad logic of this process in an invaluable book called *When Food Is Love*: "We mistake the longing to be loved and healed and valued for the longing to be thin. It's an enormous, life-altering mistake."

Roth's remark is appropriately poignant in the context of romance. But, as a Fat Chick who was duped into squandering most of her life, and all of her child-bearing years, I know there's something that must be added. The "mistake" that keeps millions of women like me from both giving and receiving love is not accidental. It's the intentional modus operandi of the weight loss industry.

9

Dumped by Design

While the antifat profiteers made a mint by piloting a mass flight from reality, various other moguls were losing their shirts. Among them was the women's apparel industry, which squandered a fortune by kowtowing to the waif-worshipping bigwigs of the fashion world. Baffled clothing execs just couldn't understand why their bottom lines were dwindling to the wispy dimensions of the gaunt models who came to dominate the mass media. But the reasons were right under their noses.

Any demographer could have told them that the skinny icons who were sashaying down the runways and cavorting on screen represented, at most, 5 percent of the female population. Any woman of average proportions would gladly have pointed out that apparel shopping was becoming more infuriating than enjoyable. And any plus-size woman who hadn't been cowed into silence would have eagerly explained why the literally slim pickings in the stores were forcing most of her clothing budget to remain unspent.

But, seduced by increasingly shrill songs touting increasingly slim sirens, manufacturers and retailers failed even to ask the pertinent questions. Instead, they meekly allowed their size ranges to stop at the point where the average American woman's body begins—and wound up spurning, by the mid-1980s, an estimated 40 million consumers with a combined buying power of $6 billion. By 1995, this total would grow to at least 50 million women, who spent an estimated $12 billion on the plus sizes that did fit them.

While influential Fifth Avenue stores were busily swapping their realistically sized mannequins for teensy Twiggy clones, no one noticed that frustrated women were scurrying out the door in droves.

Let Them Not Eat Cake

The last time anything like this had happened was back in 1947, during the now-forgotten rebellion against Christian Dior's "New Look." After centuries of wrapping, strapping, and cinching themselves to obey fashion's dictates, women had gratefully discovered comfort in the relatively relaxed clothing they wore during the Depression and the Second World War.

Suddenly, new marching orders were issued from Paris. In a radical bid to reassert the primacy of French couture after its wartime doldrums, Dior had conjured up the sort of hourglass silhouette that hadn't been seen in decades. He demanded that hemlines plunge from the knee to the ankle, that shoulder pads be shucked, and that waists be whittled by—yes, a return to corsets.

Pandemonium raged in Paris when Dior presented his first collection. Princess Elizabeth, the Duchess of Windsor, and a host of other celebrities deplored the retrogression. Across the ocean, 300,000 American women, complaining that Dior's decree "shows everything you want to hide and hides everything you want to show," formed a national protest club and vowed to resist the New Look no matter what. In just a few months, according to a *Time* cover story titled "Counter Revolution," the women's clothing industry "fell into a frightening slump."

Dior was undaunted. Even when dozens of Dallas women picketed Neiman Marcus while he was inside accepting a fashion award that autumn, he remained calm. His English may have been fractured when he opined that "I know well the women," but his prophetic prowess was right on the money: "You can never stop the fashions."

Cheered on by everyone in the clothing industry because it obliged women to scrap their entire prewar wardrobes and spend lavishly on replacements, the lucrative New Look swept to supremacy. And women obediently squashed themselves once again.

Two decades later, in the dizzying wake of Twiggymania, a similar crisis for womanly sized women occurred when de rigueur duds were rapidly downsized. This time, women wanted to comply, but the apparel industry itself made following fashion's edicts well nigh impossible for anyone who wasn't as narrow as an arrow.

It happened fast. Before miniskirts pranced onto the scene in the mid-1960s, regular clothing had routinely run to size 18 in nearly every women's store. Size 20s were frequently tacked onto the most popular lines. And for those who were even larger, half sizes were readily available, albeit generally designed with an older, not particularly fashion-conscious woman in mind.

But just a few years later, anyone larger than size 16 began to feel like a forgotten woman as she scoured the shops, boutiques, and department stores in search of fashionable clothing. Before long, the cutoff point for mass merchandise would drop to size 14 and stay that way well into the 1990s, while haute couture creations generally ran only from size 2 to size 10. Later on, someone actually came up with the most idiotic concept of all: size zero.

Some of the styles that paraded through the next three decades were absurd and some were hideous. But others—especially the sophisticated pantsuits introduced by Yves St. Laurent—were wonderful to look at and comfortable to wear, and seemed to epitomize how emancipated women wished to present themselves. Fanciful "flower child" styles gave way to the more authoritative fashions that were ideal for the millions of women who'd flooded into the workplace by the end of the 1970s, when, for the first time in history, more American women were working outside the home than remaining in it. And the need for appropriate clothing leapt exponentially, along with female purchasing power.

But size 16-and-ups were strictly wallflowers at the fashion show, forced to sit out trend after trend. Industry insiders who gave any thought at all to this sector held on to hoary assumptions that large women had little money to spend, and even less taste, and habitually postponed clothes shopping because they were perpetually planning to diet. Consequently, the options for Fat Chicks shrank to plus-size specialty chains such as Lane Bryant, smaller stores with god-awful names such as Oink Inc. and Catherine's Stout Shops, or the nether regions of department stores, where the ironically monikered "women's" departments were inevitably hidden.

Wherever large women went, the sparsity of styles was exceeded only by the dowdiness of clothes that always seemed a year or two behind the current fashions and were generally limited to cheaply produced "trailer-park" polyester. (I've never forgotten the outrageously callous answer a department store buyer gave me when I interviewed her in 1978 for a business magazine. Asked why plus-size shoppers were stuck with a plethora of polyester, she replied: "Well, they eat a lot, right? And they probably spill so much they have to keep washing their clothes. So why not give them polyester?")

Even when imitations of the most popular items from the "misses" market did turn up in large-size stores, they were usually all wrong— just ill-fitting, blown-up balloons, in pallid pastels where dark colors were called for, and vice versa, not to mention bows, ruffles, and assorted gewgaws tacked on at random by indifferent designers.

Intimate apparel was even worse. Bras and girdles were heavy, hot, industrial-strength monstrosities. Sleepwear was itchy, bulky, and often macabre enough to guarantee nightmares. Pantyhose, after taking forever to be produced in large sizes in the first place, was overpriced, yet lacked both quality and color range.

Sportswear was either too juvenile or too boisterously butch. Swimsuits were usually ugly and uncomfortably boned. Evening wear often consisted of gaudy muumuus with sequins and satin furbelows plopped in peculiar places. But the kind of attractive, high-quality, natural-fiber clothes that smaller women took for granted were nowhere to be found. All in all, plus-size choices throughout the 1970s "added up to a big yech," as a contemporary article expressed it. But the writer's timely advice—that whoever offered large women "well-made, correctly sized garments designed with some pizzazz [would] strike pay dirt"—fell on deaf ears.

How awful *was* it to shop at these establishments? Well, they did keep Fat Chicks from wandering around in gunny sacks or sewing everything we wore from scratch, so maybe we should have been grateful. But I remember peering furtively over my shoulder to make sure no one I knew was around, darting inside with the stealth and speed of a bank robber, and always making sure I had a shopping bag from some "respectable" place in which to stash the telltale plus-size sack.

To this day, a chic acquaintance of mine, who lost a lot of weight, still uses quick trips to a certain plus-size chain as "aversion therapy" to reinforce her determination to stay on the straight and narrow. And some women even celebrate their weight losses by ceremoniously cutting up their charge cards for plus-size shops.

But the worst effect for large women was that it became nearly impossible to maintain a dignified appearance—and all too easy to be perceived as the contemptible, stereotypical slobs the imagemongers insisted they were. Truth be told, human beings almost always judge books by their covers. So, as Fat Chicks were increasingly accused of having the most reprehensible covers of all—and simultaneously rendered less and less able to combat negative impressions—hostility toward them intensified as the years went by and the drumbeats of the billion-dollar brainwash grew louder.

Fashions Become Unwearable and a Plot Is Hatched

But shopping also became problematic for smaller women as the 1980s spiraled into an orgy of conscienceless consumption. The trouble was essentially that designers had become autonomous superstars, according to many observers, including Nicholas Coleridge, who points out in an eye-opening book called *The Fashion Conspiracy* that "designers like Ralph Lauren, Calvin Klein and Giorgio Armani . . . created from nothing fashion empires [that since the mid-1970s] achieved annual turnovers of $1.3, $1.1, and $1 billion respectively."

Grace Mirabella, who succeeded Diana Vreeland as editor of *Vogue*, and then founded an eponymous magazine of her own, recalls in her autobiography that "fashion came to be about nothing more than itself [and] degenerated . . . into a self-referential game full of jokes and pastiches that amused the fashion community enormously and did nothing at all for [women]."

Photographers, models, and even editors also began basking in the limelight and no longer seemed to care about anyone else's preferences or requirements. Logically, female consumers should have been in the driver's seat as never before, thanks to their new financial clout and increased need for appropriate clothing in which to pursue burgeoning employment opportunities. And certainly some designers, including Donna Karan, Liz Claiborne, and Anne Klein, were practical enough to capitalize on this situation.

But the fashion elite and the fashion press—which are, directly and indirectly, bankrolled by many of the No Fat Chicks profiteers—blithely reversed the emperor-has-no-clothes formula to an arrogant assumption that designers' creations no longer needed emperors, let alone ordinary women. As time went by, they drifted further and further into the realm of fantasy. But not the right fantasies, as far as the majority of modern women were concerned.

The zenith of this clash is generally reckoned to be the 1986 "Baby Doll" collection of French designer Christian Lacroix. In reality, the average North American woman was now thirty-two years old, weighed about 143 pounds, stood no taller than five feet four inches, and was eager for clothes reflecting her true identity. But Lacroix chose to spotlight her exact antithesis. Wobbling down the runway on teetery spike heels were towering teenage skeletons wearing ridiculously pouffed miniskirts below cinched-in bustiers, out of which their silicone-filled breasts threatened to spill. The fashion press swooned, retailers snapped up Lacroix's designs, and dress prices jumped by as much as 30 percent during the following year.

But no one had bothered to ask women if they wanted this return to what the industry called "high femininity." And no one had grasped the significance of polls indicating that—whatever their size—80 percent of women had come to detest wardrobe shopping. But women made their opinions obvious by steering clear of clothing stores during the following year and, instead, spending their money on more houses, cars, and restaurant dinners than had ever before been bought by their gender. Result: Women's apparel sales plummeted and the so-called Year of the Dress turned into a debacle.

And things just got worse as the narcissistic 1980s lurched into the nervous 1990s, and recessionary realities rocked many a boat. Profits in the regular-size clothing industry were vanishing so rapidly that designers should have done some soul-searching and asked whether, by snubbing the majority of women, they'd become their own worst enemies. Instead, encouraged by assorted antifat hucksters, they drifted so far from reality they may as well have been creating with extraterrestrials in mind.

All the over-the-top tastelessness added up to the stuff movies are made of, thought director Robert Altman, who flew his film crew to Paris in 1993 to capture the madcap collections and eccentric personalities for what later became the hilariously ironic *Ready to Wear*. Whereupon crème de la crème designer Karl Lagerfeld showed just how out of touch designers had become by fretting that the film might misportray the fashion world as "a nightmarish cartoon."

But chaos was already running amok on the runways, as increasingly tarty-looking models tottered out in sky-high skirts, slinky pants with derriere-revealing cutouts, and breasts either bared under transparent tops or clad in vulgar metallic cones. Then there were Vampira-type rubber dresses, the weird underwear-as-outerwear look, bustles, dunce caps, dog collars, and Wild West gear—and cyberspace punks decked out in a hodgepodge of clashing colors and prints. Then it was on to a tawdry parade of fake-fur skirts worn by models with multihued hair and painted-on black eyes.

None of the cynical nonsense bolstered the fashion industry's bottom line. So, in 1992, desperate designers evidently decided to try a bit of déjà vu. Crossing their fingers and hoping what worked so well in the late 1960s might get the black ink flowing again, they sent out wave after wave of gaunt waifs wearing little-girl frocks and carrying teddy bears. Sure enough, *Newsweek* dubbed the trend "Back to Twiggy." Noting that yet another scrawny English teenager was leading the pack, writer John Leland nailed the key connection: "We'd describe [Kate Moss] as four straight limbs in search of a woman's body, a mini-bosom trapped in perpetual puberty, the frail torso of the teenage choirboy—except that *Newsweek* already used this prose to describe Twiggy back in 1967."

Precisely what relevance this disinterment was meant to have for the millions of women whose age was now closer to the real Twiggy's (forty-two) than to that of little Miss Moss went unexplained. Magazine editors like *Harper's Bazaar's* Elizabeth Tilberis—who gushed that the waifs looked like "angelic little boys"—straightfacedly foisted all this bunkum on their readers and then wondered why subscriptions were sagging.

The worst was yet to come. But when it did, it was just idiotic enough to jolt retailers and manufacturers into delivering an overdue comeuppance. Swiped from the rock stars whose seedy antistyle had wafted from the mean streets of Seattle, it was aptly called the grunge look. And it consisted of little more than ragbag jeans and torn flannel shirts accessorized by scruffy sandals, greasy hair, and makeup-free faces.

Designers preened and hung $155 price tags on shirts that sold for a tenth of that at Kmart. The fashion press churned out copy hailing this exciting new "scaled-down," "reality-based" trend. But exasperated apparel moguls cut right to the chase. Exactly what part of this no-look look, they asked, can we possibly turn into socko sales? And when a fed-up flock of other marketers—representing cosmetics, jewelry, accessories, footwear, and hair products—began shouting the same cogent question, a crisis was secretly declared.

Scuttling together "like characters in an Agatha Christie novel," according to *New York Times* fashion writer Amy M. Spindler, a group of insiders set out to resuscitate profits by "deal[ing] a death blow" to the waifs and grungers. At the helm was *Vogue*'s latest editor, Anna Wintour, whose publisher talked turkey to the *Times*: "Retailers weren't moving product . . . [and] if you can't sell it, you can't advertise it."

So what *would* sell better than waifs and grungers? Glamour, glamour, and more glamour, the alleged collaborators allegedly told the finally humbled designers. Give us the works, top to bottom: fancy hair, extreme makeup, extravagant clothes, jewelry, handbags, spike heels, as many accessories as possible in between, and as much lavish lingerie as possible underneath.

All of which were duly trotted out during the spring fashion shows in 1993, even though designers had to scramble so quickly that much of the new stuff didn't make it to the stores on schedule. Not to worry. *Vogue* had it covered. Not only did the magazine take the unprecedented step of actually cofinancing some of the shows (according to Spindler), but Wintour devoted her May issue to "discovering" what she termed the switch to "Strong and Sexy." Whence had this new look "spontaneously" emanated? According to her editorial, it was inspired by women she'd seen on the streets of Paris and New York.

An ambiguous postscript was added by Tilberis when *Harper's Bazaar*, and many other publications, began going with the flow: "A lot more people will be thanking us for this look than [for] the waif." Whom she had in mind was left dangling. But one thing was clear. Nobody had bothered asking the female rank and file if skintight suits, thigh-high skirts, spike heels, waist-crushing patent leather belts, bare-it-all slip dresses, lilliputian sweater sets, daytime diamonds and sequins, garish makeup, and out-to-here hair was really what they craved.

The fashions that followed have been mostly more of the same, albeit pushing the envelope so far that *Adweek* critic Barbara Lippert has described them as "suggest[ing] prostitution, [and] sadism." And the most recent collections as of this writing featured, among other absurdities, gladiator mini-tunics, diaphanous nymph getups, barely there feather dresses, and curving goat-horn headdresses. All, according to the *Washington Post's* Robin Ghivhan, looked "so tight that not even a rivulet of perspiration would have room to roll."

Are these extremities, which include the slinky *Evita* look on which designers are currently doting, really what women want or need at this stage of the equality game? Definitely not, says Margaret Carlson, who wrote in *Time* that the hyperfeminine styles—probably best symbolized by the return of push-up bras—have a regressive subtext, especially in the employment arena: "Notice my breasts before you notice my recommendation to go long on pork-belly futures."

Fashion industry thinkers (arguably an oxymoron) could have saved themselves time, grief, and red ink, in the early 1990s and ever since, by simply checking out the *Cathy* cartoon strip drawn by Cathy Guisewite, who can always be counted on to skewer absurdities. Among many such takes on recent collections was a particularly apt panel showing an ecstatic salesclerk praising the switch to styles "designed to torture not one, not two, but every single cell of the female body!"

The Wallflowers Are Finally Asked to Dance

What was happening for Fat Chicks during this phantasmagorical frenzy? Plenty. As it turned out, there *was* life after size 14 after all. They were still being forced to sit on the sidelines watching a bewildering parade of haute couture styles that—love 'em or loathe 'em—didn't exist in their sizes. But while the regular clothing sector was foundering, aesthetically and financially, the plus-size market had begun experiencing double-digit growth. The irony was scrumptious, considering how the mainstream had so callously abandoned larger women, and that even those who did pay attention pretty much treated their customers like cheap dates they were ashamed to be seen with.

If a single person can be accorded the lion's share of the credit for wising up the apparel community, it's got to be a size-22 Californian named Carole Shaw. Sick and tired of not being able to find good clothes, she dreamed up the first American magazine for and about large ladies—*BBW: Big Beautiful Woman*—and began publishing in 1979, thus providing a national vehicle for any marketers who were savvy enough to use it. But Shaw had started raising consciousness even earlier by marching into the offices of chain store buyers and saying: "I want you to meet a fat lady in person."

The brightest of the startled buyers were all ears. They'd read a decisive demographic study (commissioned in 1978 by an international association of female clothes execs) that debunked many of the negative myths about Fat Chicks, but good. Two stats were especially eye-opening: Working women, even if they earned as little as $10,000, spent more on clothes than the nonsalaried wives of men who earned four or five times as much; and fully 37 percent of size-16-and-ups held jobs. The industry was also buzzing about the astounding success a Manhattan retailer named Nancye Radmin was having with a plus-size boutique she'd pointedly named "The Forgotten Woman." And it was beginning to dawn on the rag trade that many of the big-spending baby boomers were bound to "plump up" as they aged.

Before long, a whole gaggle of enthusiastic marketers were pursuing the very women they'd dumped nearly two decades earlier. But, observed Shaw, "it wasn't that they decided to love our big beautiful bodies. [It was that] they noticed we had that green stuff in our fat little fists."

In the vanguard among U.S. innovators were Liz Claiborne (who conferred her own first name—Elisabeth—on her large-size line), Macy's, Bloomingdale's, Saks Fifth Avenue, and The Limited, which bought Lane Bryant in 1982. And the result wasn't just burgeoning quantity, but also the quantum leap in quality that Fat Chicks had been pining for. Granted, bulletproof polyester did not die a richly deserved death. But now elegant natural fibers, in an array of flattering styles and colors, were also becoming available. *Ms.* magazine scooped its media colleagues with what it called "the garment business story of the year" in 1980. When others did finally catch on, their consensus matched the conclusion reached by the *Wall Street Journal* in 1985: "The large woman has arrived."

Gradually, other retailers and manufacturers also began taking the plunge. But they quickly bumped up against some conundrums which stymied their progress so badly that they and their predecessors probably merit an apology from yours truly and all the other Fat Chicks who maligned them for what we interpreted as disrespect.

For starters, the best designers flat out refused to risk their reputations by what they considered slumming—which was laughable, considering that Oscar de la Renta and several other biggies had happily created clothes for the Barbie doll! Gloria Vanderbilt was one of the few exceptions who didn't think catering to we-know-who would hurt her image. But even enlightened designers were daunted by the challenge of adapting their creations for bodies that were roughly double what they were used to. It wasn't as simple as just "blowing up" regular-size patterns. Proportioning was a lot trickier than that because, while small women need comparatively straight up-and-down lines, heavier bodies tend to come in either "pear" or "apple" distributions. And someone whose bust isn't all that big may have very large upper arms—a combination that makes balancing shoulders and sleeves extremely difficult.

When retailers did find designers who were willing and able to tackle all this, getting garments made could be equally tough. Manufacturers prosper by cutting in high volume. So even major players like Lane Bryant were usually forced to place their orders far in advance, yet wait for delivery until all the supposedly more profitable regular-size orders were completed. Still another problem was that, while extra fabric was obviously required, plus-size customers felt they were being gouged if prices seemed significantly higher than those paid by smaller women.

Even in the face of these stumbling blocks, however, start-up gambles soon started paying off. And a whole lot more ears began perking up when industry analysts reported that, far from being aberrant or inconsequential, the size 16-and-ups now represented at least one out of every three women in America, and 14-and-ups typified a whopping 50 percent of adult females. What really drove the point home was the fact that, while marketing myopia had kept the regular-size sector struggling, those who'd been perspicacious enough to serve Fat Chicks had shared in a market bonanza that leapt from $2 billion to $10 billion between 1982 and 1992.

Now even top designers, including Versace and Givenchy, saw the light and reached for their sketch pads. Meanwhile, upscale retailers such as Bullock's and Saks Fifth Avenue, as well as down-market giants like Kmart, J.C. Penney, Wal-Mart, and Target rushed to get in on the action. And Sears, Spiegel, and other major catalogues followed suit.

All this activity created a niche for plus-size models to exhibit the nifty new clothing in fashion shows. Specialty agencies started opening up, and such influential traditionalists as Ford and Wilhelmina gradually began recruiting large models. It took quite a while for their rotund images to start turning up in catalogues and advertisements, and there are still some surprisingly doltish holdouts (see below). But during the past two years or so, plus-size bodies modeling a wide range of clothes began appearing regularly in retail flyers, newspaper ad layouts, and a few magazines.

When a Kentucky department store chain called Bacon's took the virtually unprecedented step of choosing a plus-size model for a newspaper swimsuit ad last summer, the response was so strong that several branches had to reorder the featured suit twice during the following two weeks. And not long ago, there was another breakthrough: a series of tasteful TV commercials for Just My Size lingerie and hose featuring large-size models.

"They finally found out that we're not just housewives looking to buy a couple of blouses and a few pairs of polyester pants—we are doctors and lawyers and businesswomen," remarked Maryanne Bodolay, a coordinator for the National Association to Advance Fat Acceptance. By 1992, even Carole Shaw was almost satisfied. "I can go shopping now and find just about everything I need," she told a *Los Angeles Times* fashion writer, "but not everything I want."

Revolution Struts on Stage

Nearly everything Shaw—or any other plus-sized fashion enthusiast—could possibly wish for actually turned up two years later on a modeling runway in Toronto. It was concocted by a genuine revolutionary who is, aptly enough, named Hope—Jackqueline, or "our hero, Jackie," as she came to be known to Fat Chicks all over Canada within the span of a single decade.

The Rubenesque young woman had spent years dejectedly trudging from one store to another, searching for pretty clothes—but finding only indifference and hostility every step of the way. By the early 1980s, she'd become aware that the dismal situation was beginning to improve in the United States. But what was putting so many smiles on the faces of so many suddenly well-turned-out Fat Chicks were mostly top-down developments from industry veterans. Hope decided it was high time large women themselves started waging revolution from the grass roots up.

Their clout, as she envisioned it, would first manifest itself in looking and feeling attractive. But after reviving their own self-esteem, the long-term objective would be to set the world on a saner course—and eventually lead to restoration of the tolerance for size diversity destroyed by the billion-dollar brainwash. Hope didn't know it then but, dotted all over North America, other big women were picking themselves up, dusting off the negativity that had descended upon them since the late 1960s, and setting out in pursuit of the same ideal. (Some of their accomplishments are described in Chapter 10.)

Hope started small, "just trying to prove I was a feeling, thinking, loving, intelligent human being," while modeling for the few Canadian retailers who were taking a chance on plus-size fashion shows. She remembers "feeling very intimidated at first, like some kind of large object" that seemed to mystify audiences. Puzzled people often queried her after shows about how she could possibly have such nice-looking hair and makeup when she was so . . . uh, big. "They seemed to think there must be a different world somewhere for large people."

Stunned and stung by the assumption, Hope scraped up enough cash to rent a basement room, where she started conducting what she called "confidence seminars" for plus-size women. Even though she "didn't see anything outstanding" about herself except that she "knew how to pull it all together," she must have been doing something right. Her subterranean little business took off immediately. Word got out and she was soon invited to give motivational speeches.

Then, deciding that her solo mission to "stop any more women from shedding any more tears" would be more successful if she could also train others to be her "little soldiers," she opened a plus-size modeling agency of her own. The name: Big, Bold & Beautiful. Later, Hope and her husband added an imaginatively designed, exceptionally inviting clothing boutique, where shoppers are greeted by, not just friendly sales assistants whose girth resembles their own, but also a pair of peach-faced lovebirds whose cage sits beside a comfy couch, over which hangs a pleasing print by one of the few latter-day artists who appreciated and painted large ladies—Fernando Botero. And beside that is a TV set on which a video shows some of the shop's smashing plus-size clothes in action. On the cash counter are bright dishes filled with candies and nuts, and a stack of Big, Bold & Beautiful's sophisticated catalogues.

Above Hope's boutique, which is located in one of Toronto's trendiest areas, is the bustling agency that includes a growing stable of queen-size models. They work constantly, in the United States as well as Canada. And many of them participated in that astonishing event at Toronto's Harbour Castle Hotel in the fall of 1994. It sounds like pure fantasy from some poor schnook who's gagged down one too many diet shakes. But trust me. It really happened.

In a glitzy hotel ballroom, music suddenly begins pulsating. The lights dim dramatically. A curvaceous figure appears, nude except for a fluffy twirl of chiffon, and a knock-'em-dead fashion show hits the ground strutting. Over the next ninety minutes, a stunning succession of sumptuous clothes are paraded by an array of lovely professional models.

Enticing evening wear. Authoritative office outfits. Sprightly sports togs. Alluring lingerie. And romantic, $7,000 bridal gowns that drift dreamily to the love theme from Phantom of the Opera.

The audience goes wild. The buyers' order books are scribbled to smithereens. And the collective jaw of the fashion press drops with an audible thud. Why?

All of the models and all of the garments they wore were sizes 14 to 22.

Big, Bold & Beautiful's first major fashion show not only paid off on the promises implied in its name, but also generated the excitement it deserved. The hip VH1 channel sent a camera crew up from New York. *BBW*'s new editor, Linda Arroz (who succeeded Shaw), flew in from California and declared that she was "totally blown away." Even Fashion Television's globe-hopping Jeanne Beker covered the show.

No other plus-size marketer has so far even come close to Hope's caliber of creativity. It's the sort of special thing that seldom springs from those whose motivation is strictly monetary. It had to come from the heart and soul of a Fat Chick whose dedication was forged in a crucible of prejudice and exclusion.

But the best of the other marketers, from high-end haute to the egalitarian atmosphere at Wal-Mart, are catching on, to the extent that the number of suppliers has leapt from 200 to over 2,000 in the past seven years. The wisest among them understand why good clothes are so important, whatever one's size happens to be. As Roberta Pollack Seid defines this human imperative in *Never Too Thin: Why Women Are at War With Their Bodies*: "Dressing is . . . a process of self-creation, or self-portraiture. It reveals the way we see ourselves and the way we want others to see us. . . . We reveal our estimation of our attractiveness, of our qualities and personality traits. . . . Clothing is crucial to an individual's 'identity kit.' "

Just How Good Is It Getting?

Transformations I never expected to see, at least not until precisely one day before I checked out and headed for the Planet Rubens (my version of heaven), are turning up all over. Here are some of the highlights:

• Setting the pace for the industry, fashion consultants from Liz Claiborne's Elisabeth line have begun hosting "trunk" shows in department stores all over the country. Until this development, the opportunity to talk face-to-face with the people who control large women's shopping choices just didn't exist. The Elisabeth personnel are eager to hear customers' opinions and relay them back to the design department. And the company also sends free quarterly newsletters regarding fashion trends and tailoring improvements to anyone who requests them.

• The new "Fits Most Sizes" labels, while certainly not as good an idea as extending size ranges, are nevertheless an improvement over the fantasyland "One Size Fits All" that made so many of us feel like some kind of mutants for so long.

• Serious research is finally being done into the dimensions and proportions of a wide variety of body sizes. Spiegel, for example, before launching its excellent "For You" plus-size catalogue, meticulously measured sixteen body points, including hips, waists, busts, arms, and inseam, on a sample selection of big women. The University of Arizona also recently did what might be termed one-size-doesn't-fit-all studies on seven thousand women over age fifty-five to pinpoint what apparel alterations should be taken into consideration as women age (i.e., hips and rears often flatten, while backs may widen and chests may narrow). And a spokesperson for the American Society of Testing and Materials says that the quest to figure out what real women really look like—aimed at coming up with the same kind of standard sizing that men enjoy—is being encouraged by a great many of the apparel industry's movers and shakers.

• It's finally sinking in with designers and manufacturers that being horizontally large doesn't necessarily mean a corresponding vertical dimension. Hence a plus-size "petite" category is being developed by a lot of marketers—which comes as very welcome news to those of us who usually drown in too-long tops and are forced to wreck the lines of other garments by lopping several inches off the pants and sleeves.

• Some marketers—notably Spiegel and The Greater Woman—not only offer well-executed catalogues for home shopping, but also send fashion shows directly to customers via videos whose reasonable price (about ten dollars) can be applied toward purchases.

• Several top manufacturers of workout gear, finally acknowledging that larger women do actually exercise, have started manufacturing comfortable and functional plus-size bicycle shorts, sports bras, leotards, and other gym wear.

• Victoria can just keep her secret, because plus-size lingerie options are mushrooming, as are the inventories of gorgeously romantic unmentionables at an increasing number of shops.

• For the budget minded, or those whose weight tends to cycle at significantly different levels, plus-size consignment shops are beginning to appear.

• Just My Size and several other large-size accessories and clothing companies now have free 800 telephone numbers so that potential customers can find out the nearest location of advertised items that interest them.

• Similarly, a handful of advertisers are finally getting a clue about how to pitch to women who can spot insincerity wherever it lurks. One of my favorites is for Lee jeans, which now come in "loose" and "relaxed" fits: "Isn't it time women's clothes were designed for women? . . . How could any sane woman . . . have possibly dreamed up the bustier? What about the girdle? (Named after the sound you make when you try to put one on.)"

• The transformation of the choices available to Fat Chicks is by no means confined to North America. To name just a few other lucky locales: Many English plus-size shoppers love a London shop called 1647 whose name was chosen to emphasize the fact that 47 percent of British women wear size 16 or bigger. Large Israeli ladies are served by a store in Jerusalem called Matim Li, which, in English, means "It Suits Me." And Australia has a wide variety of chains and shops, including the upscale My Size stores in Melbourne and many other locations. Sporting what's arguably the most in-your-face name of all Down Under, there's Non-Petite, in Nelson.

• A few—make that a very few—magazines are making a conscientious effort to put a stop to the antifat madness. A special pat on the back goes to *Glamour*, which recently added a monthly page devoted mainly to plus-size fashions. Its editors also candidly reported that their art department occasionally uses computer magic to make photographed models look, not taller and thinner—as has been common for years—but larger "so that [they] don't look so anorexic."

• And best of all, in terms of their transformative potential, two new magazines, *Mode* in the United States and *Encore* in the

United Kingdom, have recently premiered. Both are pitched at women who wear size 12 and up, and both are now giving traditional women's journals a literal run for their advertising money,* and for the attention of millions of previously ignored women.

And Now for the Bad News

Apparel choices available to Fat Chicks are still far from perfect, partly, according to Alan Millstein of *Fashion Network Report*, because "[t]here is still enormous prejudice among retailers when it comes to plus sizes." After all, how much can we expect from folks who, for decades, were too dim-witted to wake up and smell the billions of dollars they were missing out on—or notice the millions of potential customers who were right under their snooty noses? Just how clueless do you have to be to keep focusing on 5 percent of your base market, while the other 95 percent are clearly doing without your stock-in-trade?

But some fashion biggies apparently are getting an inkling that there are women in the world with more meat on their bones than a couple of waifs glued together. How do we know this? Because, beginning in about 1990, they started a quiet little boondoggle that involved playing around with the numbers on the size tags. Rather than venturing into the apparently scary terra incognita beyond size 14, they simply "upsized" their garments and left the skinny little numbers in place. Upshot: "What used to be a size 8 we now call a size 6, and an 8 is what we used to call a 10," a surprisingly candid designer named Randy Kemper recently told *Glamour* magazine. Another source said that many of the most frequently used size-10 dress forms have been inflated to, on average, 36-27-38, whereas they used to be 34½-24½-34½.

There are plenty of other deserving nominees for Dolt of the Century awards. I'm sure some of their names are occurring to you even as we speak. My own include:

---

*The savviest marketers are already scrambling to buy space in *Mode*. They include Saks Fifth Avenue's Salon Z, which has never before advertised its plus-size clothing in a fashion magazine, and which, incidentally, was also perspicacious enough to furnish the TV wardrobe for talk show host Rosie O'Donnell.

• The Lane Bryant chain, which has been around longer than almost any other plus-size marketer on the planet, but still hasn't learned that "fat" isn't a synonym for "stupid." I refer, of course, to the fact that even after fairly admirable efforts to get with the Fat-Chicks-are-valuable-customers program, Lane Bryant still refuses to use large models in its catalogues. If there's a reasonable explanation for this, I was unable to elicit it in several rounds of phone tag with spokespeople in New York and Columbus. So I have no choice but to stick with the obvious explanation: They think Fat Chicks are so deluded that they believe buying these clothes will make them look exactly like the size 8s and 10s in all Lane Bryant's pretty pictures.

• Ironically, some of the most future-oriented designers of all are making the same classic mistake that cost their predecessors a fortune. Case in point: the new Levi jeans that are precisely fitted to a customer's dimensions by computer and assembled by robotic tailoring. But are these space-age britches available for the majority of female consumers? No. The size range stops where millions of women's waists begin: 35 inches.

• And, most important, because of their massive influence for good and ill, the scores of women's magazines which continue to stay in lock step with the profiteers who perpetrate the billion-dollar brainwash. Yes, of course, the major advertisers who keep them financially afloat want magazines—and movies and television and billboards—to be populated exclusively by slender, young women. But to never let a heavier, or older, woman anywhere within camera range means, by inference, telling the majority of their own readers that they don't count.

Women have put up with that sort of disrespect for centuries. But there are many signs that the days of female passivity are coming to an end. So by completely knuckling under to the bullies with the money, women's magazines are becoming less and less relevant to their readers with every passing day. And that means taking a shortcut to Dinosaurland—where all the once-mighty, now-extinct fashion moguls who wouldn't do simple math ended up.

Bottom Line

Even amidst the fury of thousands of women on both sides of the Atlantic, Christian Dior was certain that his retrogressive New Look of 1947 would soon be worn by everyone who aspired to be fashionable. His confidence proved to be well-founded, and for decades afterward, women obediently continued doing whatever designers told them to. Marching orders were, of course, delivered mostly by women's magazines—which, in turn, obeyed the big-bucks marketers who manipulated them as if they were so many marionettes.

If Dior could somehow fast-forward himself to the late 1990s, however, he'd be in for a big surprise. But it wouldn't sink in if he merely checked out what was strutting down the runways or being touted by current designers like Karl Lagerfeld, who characterized his recent collection as "elongated to death," and in magazines like *Vogue*, which recently printed a subhead the Parisian would doubtless consider flattering: "Take a deep breath. The corset and the 'waspie' waist—made popular by Christian Dior . . . in 1947—are receiving unanimous support again."

So far so good. But if Dior then strolled the streets of America and took a good look at what real women are really wearing these days, he'd have a tough time spotting *Vogue*'s purported "unanimity" about corsets, or many of the other ludicrous irrelevancies designers have tried to foist on us recently. In time, the centime would doubtless drop and the maestro would realize that the jig is just about up. As the authors of *Megatrends for Women* express it, "The days when women followed fashion blindly are over. . . . Fashion will have to start following women." Expressed even more bluntly by *Newsday*'s Denise Flaim, "Formerly trend-obsessed women are thumbing their noses at designer dictates."

As a delicious irony, and practically the only positive aspect of the thinness-above-all era, Fat Chicks have been the catalysts in the attitudinal revolution that's gradually overthrowing fashion tyrants and their handmaidens in the mass media. And the shortsighted, exclusionary dolts brought it on themselves when they deliberately prevented so many women from wearing the latest duds.

Millions tried hard—so hard that it broke many of their hearts—to whittle themselves down to what designers, marketers, and their

assorted mouthpieces told them they "should" be. But it's only a matter of time before the edict that all women should, and could, look like
the thinnest 5 percent of the female population will be exposed for the
coercive fantasy it always was. I believe the time is almost here. With
78 million baby boomers hitting middle age, the majority of buying
power is now in the hands of womanly sized women—most of whom
are old enough and wise enough to refuse to be diminished to the size,
shape, and powerlessness of waifs, baby dolls, sex kittens, or submis-
sive 1940s-style ladies.

Yet, despite the optimism prompted by this economic logic, a distinct danger still looms. The fashion industry, and the cunning marketers who keep it afloat, may simply hijack the demands of mature
women. While catering to us with more realistic sizes and styles, they
may try to exempt our daughters by continuing to hypnotize the young
into believing that the only way to be attractive is to resemble human
clothes hangers.

10

Fed Up

....

Why hasn't every window in every diet clinic in the country been smashed? Why haven't tons of pills, potions, and supplements been shoved into the Grand Canyon? Or dumpsters full of diet books, exercise videos, and fashion magazines been tossed off the Empire State Building? Why haven't the worst profiteers been sued, hanged in effigy, or force-fed some of their own noxious products? Why, in short, isn't the word "No" being screamed from coast to coast by fed-up Fat Chicks, and all the other women who feel like failures because they're not model-skinny?

Because the hardest enemy to fight is the one with outposts in your head.

The memorable aphorism from feminism's pioneer days could have no better application than this. When you're part of the only group it's still okay to hate, when your every step is dogged by condemnation, your judgment clouded by shame and guilt, your body exhausted by starvation—and you're brainwashed to blame *yourself* for all this misery—how likely is it that you'll even think of rebelling? As Naomi Wolf wrote in *The Beauty Myth*, "A quietly mad population is a tractable one."

Granted, other stigmatized groups also have to wrestle with the inner demons of doubt and fear. But the injustices faced by racial minorities, homosexuals, and the disabled are obvious to anyone who is not a bigot, and the entire culture isn't insisting that their tribulations are caused by their own character flaws—or that the solution is merely exercising sufficient willpower. For women, liberation from what Betty Friedan called "the problem that has no name" had to be generated from inside each individual's mind. But once the famous epiphanic "clicks" rose to a cacophony, the true foes were sighted and the appropriate strongholds began to be stormed.

Not so with the obese. Their stumbling block isn't that the problem has no name but that they—and everyone else—have been deliberately trained to call it by a crushing litany of wrong names: gluttony, sloth, greed, stupidity, weakness, lack of willpower, lack of self-respect, self-betrayal, antisocialism.

All of which makes it truly remarkable that, after decades of passively taking grief, a growing number of plus-size activists have finally begun dishing out some of their own. A single name for their efforts has yet to emerge, so for now, various groups characterize themselves as the size-acceptance movement, the antidiet movement, fat pride, fat power, and fat liberation. They have also been developing their own booming subculture, as we will see later in this chapter.

What did it take to motivate and embolden these Fat Chicks? Probably more than any other single factor, the overwhelming and unprecedented success of two of their own: Oprah and Roseanne. After seeing women like themselves either portrayed as inconsequential buffoons or being invisible altogether, watching these two role models achieve mogul status, on their own terms, has been enormously empowering. (And subsequent weight losses by both women did nothing to diminish the effect.)

The Go button was also punched by the discovery of exonerating medical evidence that obesity is not caused or perpetuated by simply eating too much. Not only have "fat genes" been discovered, but the counterproductivity of dieting is now incontestable. So when Fat Chicks insist that they're not gorging themselves, that their metabolisms have been wrecked by dieting, and that it's impossible for 95–98 percent of all dieters to sustain weight loss, they know they're telling truths that are finally beginning to be believed.

The breathtakingly cruel depths to which antifat profiteers have recently sunk has acted as a third motivator. When, for example, *Harper's Bazaar* magazine virtually endorsed the potentially lethal scourge of bulimia as a normal beauty imperative, hackles were raised all over the continent. Sympathy for Princess Diana was widely expressed when, directly following her admission that she had suffered severe bulimia, she was hounded about her appearance in a much-repeated Reuters "news" story reporting that she had taken to wearing long coats to conceal cellulite on her thighs. And one of the worst flops in fashion history occurred when what might be termed Operation Waif (actually Twiggy Revisited) tried to convince women that the new standard of beauty was epitomized by emaciated teenage girls who looked as if they needed rescuing from prisoner-of-war camps.

That the attitudinal tide is starting to turn—and not just among Fat Chicks—was recently demonstrated by an unprecedented, evidently spontaneous, graffiti campaign that recently defaced dozens of Calvin Klein jeans ads featuring "superwaif" model Kate Moss. Across her concave bare stomach were scrawled variations on the theme of "Feed this woman." And beside her droopy mouth, cartoon-type balloons appeared, saying, "I'm so hungry!" Irate mothers of "waif wannabes" also protested this ad campaign by mailing jeans back to Calvin Klein with blistering comments about his irresponsible attitude.

Comes the Revolution

Radicalized by these events and similar factors, size-acceptance advocates are being galvanized into action by adding up the numbers and realizing their potential clout—economic, political, and, ultimately, social. When you figure in not only the truly overweight, but also the millions of women who are coerced into everlasting diets despite being average or even underweight, their numbers dwarf those of all other shortchanged groups combined. Tallying up the numbers reveals a horrifying total of well over 100 million American women who are affected and afflicted by the billion-dollar brainwash.

Small wonder, then, that those in the vanguard of the size-acceptance movement insist their efforts represent the next cultural transformation. And that once the majority of Fat Chicks, and those who identify with them, finally comprehend the enormity of the disservice that's being done—not only to women of all sizes, but to yet another generation of girls—the revolution will be unstoppable.

Considering their collective purchasing power, plus the fact that their ranks include an estimated 80 percent of the 78 million big-spending American baby boomers, who become chunkier rather than scrawnier as they age—and therefore are more than likely to revamp injustices in this context, just as they've done in so many other arenas—simple logic suggests just one outcome: It's only a matter of time before fat people will stop being the only minority it's still socially acceptable to laugh at and discriminate against.

No one thinks it's going to be easy. But it *is* starting to get interesting. Size-acceptance crusaders say they have the heady feeling that their struggle is approaching the stage where it can be legitimately compared with the early days of the civil rights and women's liberation movements. And the same general plot outline does indeed seem to be unfolding. The fight is proceeding amid identical derision from reactionary observers. And the attitudinal first step has been taken, which is reclaiming the adjective that's used as the sharpest weapon of oppression. For African Americans it was "black," and in this context, of course, it is "fat."*

Recently, there were unmistakable echoes of earlier insurrections when the most prominent group of (primarily) Fat Chicks went on the offensive—by taking the battle out of their own heads and into the streets.

They chose the favorite tactic of all revolutionaries who want to symbolize their determination to overcome: a march on the capital. Near a spot in Washington, D.C., where Martin Luther King once appealed for racial equality, demonstrators from the National Association to Advance Fat Acceptance (NAAFA) marked their twenty-fifth anniversary, on August 26, 1994, by declaring their own dream: "To be treated like human beings."

The poignancy of the plea reflected the sheer courage it had taken for most of the portly protesters just to show up. Like the women's liberationists, African Americans, and homosexuals who preceded them down Pennsylvania Avenue years ago, these activists knew that their mere appearance would be inflammatory. But this time, it was bound

---

*This is why I chose to use the insulting term "Fat Chicks" as the title of this book, and to repeat it until it has been robbed of its hurtful power.

to be worse. When you can't even step outside your door without attracting catcalls, you know that parading your despised body means deliberately venturing into harm's way.

The fear was well-founded, and it didn't take long for the insults to come flying on that sweltering summer day. As undermining as it undoubtedly was for earlier protesters to hear racial and sexual epithets, or to see placards ordering women back to the kitchen, it was an infinitely more personal humiliation to have to stare down placards shrieking: "Save a Whale—Harpoon a Fat Chick!"

But the gutsy demonstrators refused to be intimidated by the naked prejudice they endured during their march, or the demeaning media coverage by the few news organizations that paid attention. Typical was Gannett News Service's Carl Weiser, who facetiously estimated that the protesters "were burning off 300 calories an hour," and then dismissed the event by adding that "government has become a veritable food fight of special interests, leaving democracy paralyzed by a barrage of incoming vegetables."

While Weiser's unwieldy metaphor made little sense, the *Los Angeles Times*'s Scott Harris missed the point altogether. Sticking to the standard media approach of trying to sniff out dissension, he wound up his article about the size-acceptance movement with what he apparently thought was a humorous kicker. NAAFA executive director Sally E. Smith, Harris wrote, had "grumbled [that] the closest [she'd] come to killing a talk show guest" was when she shared a stage at the *Leeza* TV show with *Diary of a Fat Housewife* author Rosemary Green, who repeated her frequently expressed opinion that "big is not beautiful. It's ugly and disgusting."

The blatancy and prevalence of such insults explain why it took a quarter century after the founding of NAAFA just to get this far. Despite an increasingly overweight American populace, membership in what is, so far, the only viable fight-back organization on the continent stands at a meager 4,500. But then, as NAAFAns reassure one another, it took nearly fifty years after winning the vote in 1920 for women to raise enough consciousness to start rewriting the rules that diminished them—and about the same gap after its 1909 founding before the National Association for the Advancement of Colored People (NAACP) grew strong enough to begin righting racial wrongs.

Yet some commentators vehemently object to comparing the size-acceptance crusade to the civil rights movement. "Ridiculous," said David Boaz, executive vice president of the libertarian Cato Institute, when queried about a recent successful lawsuit launched by a 360-pound Tennessee woman named Deborah Birdwell against a Nashville cinema that refused to allow her to bring in her own folding chair, despite the fact that its seats could not accommodate her. "Trivializing," echoed Kansas City based political movement authority Laird Wilcox, who provided an object lesson by opining in a syndicated article that NAAFA's efforts are merely "silly [because] people prefer to be around those who are attractive, not unattractive."

Even more inimical to the size-acceptance struggle for credibility, given that it appeared in one of the most influential of all magazines, was an uncharacteristically thoughtless *Time* essay by Margaret Carlson. After a breezy beginning—"Got a weight problem? . . . phone Uncle Sam . . . and you could get a wad of cash or that job you've been wanting"—the piece, titled "And Now, Obesity Rights," deplored the exemplary legal victories of two large women whose employment discrimination was discussed in Chapter 6.*

Carlson concluded her shortsighted essay by warning that to include fat people in protective legislation would be "to fail . . . the truly vulnerable, the truly prejudged, the truly disadvantaged." But it's the firm conviction of size-acceptance proponents that they *do* belong in these negative categories that is fueling the increasingly feisty efforts.

As the primary force in the size liberation movement, NAAFA has come a long way since its 1969 founding, when newsletters were sent out in plain brown envelopes to avoid embarrassing members. But the group's philosophy—that no one should have to be thin to enjoy the same rights and privileges due every other citizen—has never changed. Ongoing consciousness-raising activities by various NAAFA committees include lobbying lawmakers (see below), the medical community,

---

*But, in the case of Bonnie Cook, the nursing aide who prevailed in court against a Rhode Island mental-retardation facility, Carlson (and many other journalists) left out some crucial information. The 320-pound Cook had *already* performed her duties satisfactorily at the same facility for three years, before a daughter's illness forced her to resign. Yet when she reapplied for her old job, weighing exactly the same amount as before, she was turned down because of obesity.

advertisers, educators, housing authorities, airlines, film producers, and other industries. Media appearances by executive director Sally E. Smith and vigorous letter-writing campaigns by members have resulted in the sensitization of many (although obviously not enough) editors and news directors. One of Smith's personal bests to date, in terms of exposure for her cause, was convincing *USA Today* to publish her hard-hitting, advertiser-offending piece titled "The Great Diet Deception" in January 1995. Smith has also hit the lecture circuit, speaking to, among other crucial sectors, medical students and those who teach them. In addition, NAAFA's board of directors includes an impressive, influential, and exceptionally active group of health professionals.

Other activist organizations and individuals currently are working to undo the damage done by the billion-dollar brainwash:

• A-HELP (Association for the Health Enrichment of Large People), an organization of professionals in the medical, mental health, health education, and scientific communities who share the belief that "fat" and "fit" are not mutually exclusive terms. In addition to sponsoring seminars and other consciousness-raising events, A-HELP members frequently publish articles such as a recent one in *Radiance* magazine by Joanne Ikeda, R.D., titled "Confessions of a Radical Registered Dietician."

• In Santa Cruz, California, the Body Image Task Force has tackled the need for theatres to provide extra-wide seats and, at this writing, was negotiating with both the United Artists and Harris Group movie chains.

• In Dallas, Texas, a group of women with a raucous sense of humor publishes a consciousness-raising magazine called *Rump Parliament*. They also confer annual Rumpie Awards on those who "perpetuate negative stereotypes about fat people." Columnist Ann Landers, for example, recently received a Rumpie in the category of "Broken Record" for, said the citation, her "insistence on using that tired phrase 'killing yourself with a knife and fork.'" Although Landers expressed ambivalence about the accusation, she good-naturedly gave the organization a quantum leap by featuring it in her column.

• Dedicated to furthering the antidiet philosophy among clients and other health professionals, Hugs International is a Canadian company with facilitators in four other countries, including the United States. Founder Linda Omichinski, R.D., is the author of a bestseller, *Calories Don't Count, You Do*, and coauthor of a companion book, *Tailoring Your Tastes*. She also publishes a newsletter and distributes video and audio cassettes "to help people move from dieting to focusing, instead, on health and energy."

• In addition, a growing number of smaller self-help organizations are springing up all over the continent. These include Breaking Free workshops conducted by author Geneen Roth (whose invaluable books I've gratefully borrowed from throughout *No Fat Chicks*); Great Shape and New Face of Fitness classes designed specifically for heavy women; and the Beyond Hunger and Overcoming Overeating groups, both of which teach their members how to stop dieting and relearn their natural appetites.

International No-Diet Day

Staged annually on May 5 for the past several years in various cities in England and Australia, International No-Diet Day was imported into North America about five years ago, largely through the efforts of *Rump Parliament* editor/publisher Lee Martindale. The object is to stage events to encourage fat people to publicly raise consciousness by picketing diet centers and weight-loss-surgery establishments, feeding the hungry, and enjoying guilt-free meals (such as mass picnics) themselves. Martindale's scheme got a big boost when Ann Richards, then the governor of Texas, proclaimed No-Diet Day in her state in 1994.

Regional wrinkles are being added by NAAFA members like Ron Karle, a computer programmer in Ann Arbor, Michigan, who mobilizes fitness walks for obese people "to show that we can exercise too, and that we have the right to use public parks without being ridiculed." Elsewhere, NAAFAns in Seattle and San Diego have held public smashings of bathroom scales and marched under such banner slogans as "Scales Are for Fish, Not Women." And another feisty group, in Edmonton, Canada, dreamed up a hilarious death-for-dieting demonstration, complete with a jazzy New Orleans-style funeral procession and a coffin into which were tossed dozens of weight loss items they deemed "toxic."

New York City's National Center for Overcoming Overeating has sponsored a Diet Museum featuring outrageously useless and exploitive artifacts, while a huge picnic was held in Portland, Connecticut. And in Woodstock, New York, two activist groups—Substantial Women and the Fat Feminist Caucus of NAAFA—sponsored a recent exhibit called "Women Artists Celebrate Fat Women."

At this writing, there has been talk, but no action, regarding more radical ideas for celebrating International No-Diet Day. Example: "bombing" diet centers with exploding bags of ketchup to dramatize the fact that the H. J. Heinz food company, which owns Weight Watchers, nabs consumers coming and going—by first tempting us to gain weight with saturation-level advertising of its food products, and then signing us up for reducing classes, as well as selling us expensive items from its burgeoning repertoire of low- and no-fat products.

If such extreme tactics *are* ever exercised by some future guerilla organization, its members may gain inspiration from the consciousness-raising antics of a gutsy group that no longer exists. It was called the Fat Underground, and it waged psychological war on a host of antifat profiteers in the mid-1970s. The death of singer Mama Cass Elliot—and especially its false attribution to overeating (see Chapter 11)—galvanized the troupe. From more tepid activities, they revved up to employing confrontational tactics that included sponsoring a Women's Day rally in Los Angeles at which they accused the diet industry of having murdered Elliot. Later, the Fat Underground began invading Weight Watchers classes and other such meetings, blocking the exits, seizing the microphones to harangue people with the truth about punitive dieting, and then making rapid getaways in waiting cars.

Consumer Boycotts

How about the ultimate fight-back tactic of any protest movement: the consumer boycott? NAAFA recently organized a boycott of Hallmark that persuaded the company to drop an offensive line of greeting cards, mugs, and other items that made fat people the butt of their dubious humor. (Sample: An elephant in a hammock above the quote "I exer-

cise as much as the next guy—provided the next guy is a fat, lazy slob!")
In addition, NAAFA's threat of calling a boycott of the Denny's restaurant chain—because much of its seating is too small—succeeded in
eliciting a pledge to correct the situation in all future restaurants.

In Boston in early 1994, a group called Boycott Anorexic Marketing
(BAM) began targeting companies whose advertisements feature
extremely thin models. Psychotherapist and eating-disorders specialist
Mary Baure says she helped facilitate the group's formation because "so
many women [feel] powerless at the way our culture applauds anorexia."
High on BAM's hit list are Calvin Klein, for those notorious Kate Moss
jeans ads, and a Coca-Cola product called Diet Sprite, because of its use
of a skin-and-bones model named Kristin McMenamy, whom the print
ad nicknamed "Skeleton." Although Coca-Cola officially denied any
backlash from BAM's activities, the ad was canceled.

The group's power and visibility were enormously enhanced when
the National Organization for Women endorsed its efforts in May
1994. Said NOW's Los Angeles chapter president, "Advertising has
always been used to impact our society's way of thinking, and women
have been paying the price for far too long."

Setting Watchdogs on the Profiteers

Several victories for size-acceptance activists have occurred since 1990,
when Senator Ron Wyden, a Democrat from Oregon, declaring that
"[m]illions of Americans abused by this industry may as well burn their
money on the curb for all the good they get," and convened congressional hearings on the weight loss industry. Before the final gavel
pounded, several governmental bodies—the Food and Drug Administration (FDA), the Federal Trade Commission (FTC), the Federal
Communications Commission (FCC), and the Attorney General's
Office—were officially blasted for letting things get so out of hand by
failing to investigate abuses or even to enforce existing regulations.

In a whirlwind of subsequent actions, the FTC commenced a three-
year investigation that ended up charging five of the nation's largest
commercial diet programs—including Weight Watchers, Jenny Craig,
and Nutri/System—with deceptive advertising practices. By the end of
1994, when the dust had cleared, Weight Watchers' membership had

plunged by between 15 and 25 percent (depending on which news report you believe). Nutri/System declared bankruptcy and closed its 283 centers (but metamorphosed eight months later into a "wellness" program). And Jenny Craig, which put up a fair bit of resistance, ended up with its stock at an all-time low and a 19 percent revenue drop, forcing it to close about thirty branches. Also, Jenny Craig paid out $10 million to settle a class-action suit on behalf of customers who accused it of misleading advertising and medically unsafe practices.

The FDA has investigated and banned 111 ingredients from over-the-counter pills, ruling them ineffective or potentially harmful, and cracked down on a wide range of products. At least six product-liability suits have been filed against Medifast (including charges that the program causes gallstones and gangrene).

Meanwhile, the FTC began hounding many of the worst profiteers regarding the safety and efficacy of their products and the grandiosity of their assertions. A ubiquitous pill called Fibre Trim was put out of business altogether while, at this writing, a similar fate seemed to be facing such other snake oil products as FormulaTrim 3000, Megaloss 1000, and MiracleTrim. But the most significant result of all was an edict that such disclosure statements as "For many dieters, weight loss is temporary" must be added to some product packaging, and to all broadcast ads of more than thirty seconds' duration.

After considering a report by a panel of experts it commissioned in 1994, the Washington-based Institute of Medicine issued a fairly well-publicized statement urging the weight loss industry "to disclose the true effectiveness of its programs" and to consider establishing an accreditation process.

Have all these efforts made much of a difference to the prosperity of the billion-dollar brainwash so far? Not really. But they *are* a laudable beginning.

As for the future, NAAFA, which has done the lion's share of consumer lobbying, is now calling for the following steps: that the U.S. Centers for Disease Control and Prevention start tracking the incidence of deaths related to weight loss efforts; that the ban keeping tobacco advertising off radio and television be extended to include dangerous diet products; and that the Surgeon General begin requiring that all weight loss products carry a warning about their probable ineffectiveness, similar to the cautionary messages now mandatory for all cigarette packaging.

Project Legislation 2000 is another program that's under way, with ad hoc support from several activist groups. Its goal is to have the words "weight or size" added to existing antidiscrimination legislation by the turn of the century in all of the states where they are currently absent.

And finally, spurred by the premise that to change the future, it's essential to change the attitudes of the young people who will inherit it, the Human and Civil Rights Division of the (U.S.) National Education Association is currently investigating size discrimination in public schools.

A Rising Subculture

Civil rights leader Malcolm X often spoke about how demoralizing it is to never see anyone who resembles you portrayed as a normal participant in popular culture. He meant African Americans, of course, but large women have been marginalized in exactly the same way since the billion-dollar brainwash shifted into high gear in the late 1960s.

Not content to simply wait for readmission into the mainstream, the boldest and most entrepreneurial of the Fat Chicks are developing a burgeoning subculture all their own. Besides the proliferation of plus-size clothing and modeling agencies detailed in Chapter 9, there are social clubs with defiant names such as "Goddesses" and "More to Love," which range from supportive all-female get-togethers to dance parties which provide a comfortable atmosphere in which to meet men who appreciate fat women despite—or because of—their size.

There are religious groups, swimming parties, and even cruises and other vacation trips exclusively for overweight people. There are hair stylists, photographers, psychotherapists, cosmeticians, dieticians, exercise classes, fitness trainers, massage therapists, and even bankers who specialize in large-size clients.

There are also dozens of mail-order catalogues, with names like "Royal Resources," "Far and Wide" and "Amplestuff," that feature clothing, books, video and audio tapes, personal-care items (such as extra-size clothes hangers, tape measures, and hospital gowns), and posters like one that advertised a recent "vision-expanding" photographic exhibition called "The Belly Project." Among the most popular of the inspirational items aimed at size-acceptance proponents are replicas of the 30,000-year-old Woman from Willendorf, which is the oldest known "Earth Mother" statue. Her rotund image is being reproduced as jewelry, art objects, and even chocolates. Other hot items include T-shirts sporting such slogans as: "A waist is a terrible thing to mind," and "If this were the 1500s, I'd be a goddess!"

Fat Chicks have their own magazines, which not only feature flattering pictorial coverage of large women modeling attractive clothing, but also provide a forum for their stories, relevant news, pertinent articles, and resource indexes. The first of these publications was *BBW: Big Beautiful Woman*, which began in 1979. Also popular are *Dimensions*, which includes a very active dating-service feature to introduce large women to men who admire them; and *Mirage*, which works the other way around by publishing photographs of male "fat admirers" who are interested in meeting heavy women. Two excellent sources of unbiased information about up-to-the-minute obesity research are the *Healthy Weight Journal* and NAAFA's newsletter.

The best of the bunch may turn out to be *Mode*, which had just debuted as of this writing. For now, however, it is definitely *Radiance*, which has been published out of Oakland, California, for the past eleven years. A lively quarterly that's reminiscent of *Ms.* in its early days, the magazine occasionally engages in good-naturedly radical tactics such as publishing a swimsuit edition that puts *Sports Illustrated*'s obnoxious equivalent to shame. *Radiance* also features unique and extremely useful articles (sample: "How to Cope With Anti-Fat Doctors"), plus an investigative column by NAAFA cofounder William J. Fabrey called "Big News," and a regular medical column by biomedical researcher Dr. Paul Ernsberger on vital topics such as the risks involved in weight loss surgery.

The bold spirit of the size-acceptance movement in general, and *Radiance* in particular, was recently expressed in a punchy editorial by the magazine's founder and publisher, Alice Ansfield, who warned: "Watch out, thin people, we fatties are coming out. We're not going to stay safely in our homes anymore, so you'd better get used to it."

Media Coverage

Are the media catching on to the sensational story that's right under their noses? In most cases, the answer is no. And some of the pundits who are wising up to the size-acceptance revolution still resemble the proverbial blind folk trying to discern the outline of an elephant and misidentifying the parts they do manage to grasp.

Boston Globe columnist Diane White, for example, recently wrote a sarcastic piece trivializing discrimination against overweight women. NAAFA's Sally Smith objected in a published letter, saying that White had "reinforc[ed] myths and negative stereotypes about fat people." Whereupon White—while describing herself as a large woman—compounded her offense by writing a second column dismissing Smith's complaint. Her tone was an all-too-familiar winking at readers, as if to say, "We all know that fat people are fair game, so let's have at it."

And when *No Fat Chicks* was released in Canada recently, a newspaper headlined an article about my book: "Ugly Fattie Weighs in Against Bulge Battle."

There are, however, a growing number of writers and broadcasters who *are* beginning to sense something new in the wind. Television shows such as *Prime Time Live* and *20/20* have broadcast, respectively, a shocking exposé of the latest—and potentially most dangerous—type of weight loss surgery, and on the growing "fat but fit" movement.

Several of the most influential American publications have begun exploring the same theme. *People*, for example, using a phrase that's become almost extinct, urged "superwaif" model Kate Moss to "put some meat on her bones." In another issue, *People* put Moss on its cover beside the words: "Skin & Bones: . . . Is a dangerous message being sent to weight-obsessed teens?" The magazine also regularly features 155-pound Guess jeans model Anna Nicole Smith, and included a 180-pound plus-size model named Emme in a recent compilation of "The 50 Most Beautiful People." Emme is also the first plus-size model to appear on one of Times Square's giant billboards in New York City. Certainly these items fall in the "fluff" category, but the routine inclusion of large women in such popular coverage is a vital part of what's being striven for by size-acceptance advocates.

On a more serious note, *Ladies' Home Journal* editor Leslie Lampert took the dramatic step of having a realistic "fat suit" designed by theatrical costumers to let her pass for a woman of about 250 pounds as she pursued a week of normal activities in New York City. In an admirably eye-opening article titled "Fat Like Me," Lampert described not only the outward cruelty and discrimination she experienced while wearing her disguise, but also the inward depression such treatment fostered. "I feel ashamed of my culture," Lampert concluded, "[for the] pain we cause people who are less than our concept of ideal."

Three circulation giants, *Reader's Digest, Consumer Reports,* and *USA Weekend,* carried the very positive "don't diet—be happy" message of Martin E. P. Seligman's inspirational best-seller *What You Can Change and What You Can't* to millions of readers who might otherwise not have discovered the book. *USA Weekend* also published an excellent report on the antidiet revolution by Jacqueline Shannon titled "New Research: Fat Isn't Voluntary"; and its weekly "Fitness With Foreman & Flo-Jo" column also deserves commendation for a no-nonsense philosophy epitomized recently by Olympic athlete Florence Griffith Joyner in her answer to a reader's query: "You can't tell a person's fitness level by his appearance," she wrote. "It doesn't matter if you're 95 pounds or 300 pounds; what matters is being fit."

Far ahead of the pack is *Psychology Today*, especially for a cover story reporting the results of its 1997 Body Image Survey (January/February issue)—which irrefutably documents the devastation created by the billion-dollar brainwash.

Among the most widely circulated women's magazines, a sort of schizophrenic identity crisis has recently been in evidence. Even while sprinkling their issues with dump-your-diet articles, they're still filling the remaining pages with photos of extremely thin women. The May 1995 *Vogue* was typical. Tucked into a waif-strewn issue that editor Anna Wintour inexplicably touted as "the first ever devoted to the body" was a top-notch investigative piece by Laura Fraser.* Entitled "Dieting by Prescription," it cast a merciless eye on the recent resurgence of diet medications. Fraser, who candidly described herself as

*Fraser is the author of *Losing It: America's Obsession with Weight and the Industry That Feeds on It*, from which I have gratefully gleaned important information.

weighing "a robust 155 pounds," first wangled her way into a profit-making seminar at a convention of the American Society of Bariatric Physicians, and later posed as a potential patient in the offices of a variety of pill-pushing doctors. Summing up, she said that she "became enraged thinking about all the people who trust their doctors to help them with a problem, pay them a lot of money, dutifully starve themselves, then blame themselves when they've gained the weight back."

Bottom Line

"The forfeited self" is an eloquent term Betty Friedan coined in *The Feminine Mystique* to characterize what women lost during the materialism-dominated decades immediately after the Second World War. But the label applies equally well to those who've been most damaged by the billion-dollar brainwash. So does Friedan's formula for defeating oppression: "Refuse to be nameless, depersonalized, manipulated, and live [your] own lives again according to self-chosen purposes."

We certainly won't enter the twenty-first century entirely liberated from the No Fat Chicks commandment. But size-acceptance and anti-diet activists are walking, talking, shouting, singing, scale-smashing demonstrations of what happens when the mental penny drops and Fat Chicks finally understand the enormity of what has been done to them—and what must be done to stop it.

The wisest of the protesters perceive the parallels with other oppressed groups and are borrowing vital strategic techniques from earlier revolutionaries. They firmly believe that if their battle is fought on behalf of, and in solidarity with, every person of every size and circumstance who's ever been hurt by discriminatory commercial and cultural factions, they *will* overcome some day.

11

Dying to Be Thin

Of all the people I've ever written about, the only one who haunts me is a woman I never met. Her name was Juliette Christie, and she'd been dead for six months by the time I began investigating how her lifelong obsession with losing weight killed her.

It was the autumn of 1981, and I was teetering at the halfway point in my own "diet to end all diets." Coast to coast, I was being cheered on by thousands of women who read my magazine diary, identified with my struggle, and believed in its goal as unquestioningly as I did. But the pounds weren't coming off fast enough to hit my deadline, and I had begun to think I was headed for disaster. Then the phone rang and the editor of another magazine asked me to write an article about Juliette's death.

I knew I shouldn't do it, because my diet series was taking every ounce of time, energy, and courage I could scrape together. But I said yes anyway, telling myself it was because this was a plum assignment that could boost my writing career. And that I was bound to do a good job because I could bring a great deal of expertise to the story. But that wasn't the reason.

The truth was so brutal I've never admitted it until now. What really motivated me to tackle Juliette's story was the same compulsion that drove me to a circus sideshow when I was a teenager. I thought I should force myself to stare at the Fat Lady. I thought

204

looking at her as if she were a mirror reflecting my own disgusting image was the punishment I deserved for being overweight. I hoped this do-it-yourself shock therapy might jolt me into finally getting rid of my excess pounds. And most of all, I prayed that performing this humiliating penance would buy me redemption for the sin I had evidently committed.

There were just the two of us in the musty tent that day. The Fat Lady sat on a platform about six feet from the makeshift fence that separated us. She glanced at me for a brief moment with no change in expression, no flicker of the filial recognition I'd been expecting. Then she silently dismissed me and gazed impassively toward something I couldn't see.

My pathetic little pilgrimage didn't work. When I looked at the Fat Lady, I couldn't see myself after all. In fact, I couldn't see anyone inside that massive barrel of flesh. She wouldn't let me—any more than Juliette would, years later. She was dead. And maybe I'd be joining her soon, at the rate I was going.

At least that's how I felt as I sat through a coroner's inquest, exhausted, heartbroken, hungry, and frightened by the familiarity of what I was hearing. But these feelings would soon be compounded by dismay at an outcome that failed to draw the obvious conclusion: society's hatred can be lethal.

None of the testimony about her was very personal. But somehow I gathered that Juliette wasn't much of a reader, and probably never knew the legend of Sisyphus. Yet for much of her miserably conflicted life, she was trapped in just such a classic struggle. Fat was her rock— one hundred pounds too much of it by the end—and the mountain was her own obstinate body. No matter how hard she tried, how stoically she denied her appetite, or even how successful she was—more than once accomplishing heroic losses of over fifty pounds—her burden always came rolling back. And along with it, the anguish of belonging to the one group it's still all right to mock, despise, and discriminate against.

As clear a symbol as the skull and crossbones on a bottle of poison, Juliette collapsed and died on the doorstep of a weight loss center. Flat on her back in a pool of vomit as an exhausted heart surrendered on her behalf, she became another of the untold, unmourned casualties of a deadly scourge it would take me fifteen more years to recognize as the billion-dollar brainwash.

The day she died, four days short of her fifty-seventh birthday, Juliette had a family who loved her, and she was under the care of a fully qualified physician and a reputable pharmacist. But she was en route to yet another appointment with yet another antifat profiteer. It happened to be a branch of the (now defunct) Weight Loss Clinics of America. But it could have been any of the temples of corporeal salvation that have mushroomed ever since our society was conned into fixating on the image of an emaciated teenage model.

It seems dreadfully significant, however, that the Weight Loss Clinic's head office was located in a narcissistic community like Marina Del Rey, California. Halfway between the frenzy of LAX and the phony paradise of Venice, it was about three thousand miles away from the lobby where Juliette died. Yet its stock-in-trade was powerful enough to leap the geographic and socioeconomic gulf that, logically, should have prevented the emotional enslavement of a middle-aged Canadian matron.

But logic played as minor a role in this story as it does in the ongoing ordeals of millions of other women who try so hard to achieve the impossible. And Juliette's obsession with conforming to her culture's artificially manipulated aesthetic standards made her just as vulnerable as the Haitian refugees who were then in the headlines for risking everything aboard another type of manifestly dubious vessel. Their bodies were washing ashore in Florida at about the same time Juliette's inquest concluded in Toronto.

By then I knew a lot about how she died. But exactly what kept her trapped in jeopardy at that mature a stage of life still eluded me. "The biggest question," I wrote, "[must] remain unanswered:

> How could she have reached ostensible maturity, successfully raised a loving daughter, lived to enjoy two grandchildren, maintained a reportedly happy relationship with her husband and a job she loved, and still be controlled by a compulsion that most women in her position would, surely to God, have felt fulfilled enough to abandon decades earlier?

It Must Be Worth It

The beginning of the end for Juliette was her decision—after a lifetime of dieting—to put herself in the hands of the nice nurses who staffed the local branch of Weight Loss Clinic. She weighed 251 pounds, which she told them she knew was at least 100 pounds too much for her five-foot, five-inch frame. But, as a beginning, her short-term goal was to knock off 50 pounds in time for a family reunion on her birthday, which was just four months away. Would this be possible?

No problem, the nurses assured her. Yet achieving such a large loss so rapidly would require a whopping deficit of nearly 1,500 calories every single day—by someone who was nearly sixty years old, had a dismal track record, was known to crave sweets, and whose only physical exercise consisted of a gentle aquatic routine once in a blue moon. Mind you, she did exert herself prodigiously on her job as a Red Cross homemaker, tending to the personal and practical needs of the elderly and chronically ill, and frequently going beyond the call of duty by scrubbing their walls and floors.

Juliette's salary for this was barely above minimum wage, and her elderly husband brought in only a military veteran's pension. Yet she somehow came up with the Weight Loss Clinic fee of $626.40. Later on, when her daughter became alarmed enough about her condition to urge her to give up the diet, Juliette said (in her native French so that her husband wouldn't understand), "Are you kidding? Your dad would kill me if I spent all that money and didn't lose the weight."

This was far from the truth. It showed, rather, that the clinic's steep fees were more of an inducement than a repellent for Juliette, who seemed to be one of the many people who are predisposed to the notion that if something costs an outrageous amount of money, it *must* be worth it. Which explains why the majority of the antifat scammers' most blatantly exploitative articles and advertisements appear in the media vehicles pitched to people with the least education and sophistication. (See any issue of any supermarket tabloid for such obvious examples as Jenny Craig's advice column in *The National Enquirer*.)

The Weight Loss Clinic's staff didn't just grab Juliette's check with no questions asked. They took her blood pressure, just as they would do every week until she died, and found it acceptable. Later, when questioned at the inquest as to whether they always used a large-size blood pressure cuff on her fat upper arm, they insisted they had. But a medical expert testified that the final few readings before Juliette's death were so rock-bottom they could have been produced "only by a healthy teenager." Yet the nice nurses had seen no cause for doubt.

Nor, at the outset, had they been concerned about Juliette's negative medical history, which included gallbladder disease, hypertension, recurring gout, and shortness of breath. Or the daily diuretics she said she was taking for her gout, even though these are known to rob the body of vital elements such as potassium. None of these factors discouraged the nurses from putting Juliette on the clinic's second-most-rigorous program—a scant 800 calories a day.

What they didn't know about—because Juliette was so desperate to lose weight that she lied—were the many other medications she was taking, which caused her to be characterized at the inquest as "a walking drugstore." Hidden at the back of her breadbox, and discovered by her daughter after Juliette's death, were appetite suppressants, antidepressants, Tylenol, tetracycline, and antihistamines. Almost all had been prescribed by her regular physician and provided by a neighborhood pharmacist who knew Juliette well enough to testify that he "just knew something like this was going to happen sooner or later."

The Weight Loss Clinic had no physician on staff or on call—just the endorsement of psychologist Joyce Brothers, whose smiling image was then appearing in numerous print and TV ads. Usually, she was photographed reading a letter which was ostensibly from yet another satisfied customer. "Dear Dr. Brothers, I can't tell you what it means to be able to wear short white shorts in public."

No one knew if Juliette was attracted to the Weight Loss Clinic by one of these ads. But when her physician—who happened to be a fairly recent immigrant from Guyana and apparently didn't know Dr. Brothers from Dr. Seuss—took the stand, she was asked whether she had believed the clinic's medical supervision was sufficiently safe to allow her patient to follow the strict regimen. "Well, yes," she said. "It's in all the advertisements. It's Dr. Joyce Brothers."

So Juliette's doctor confidently okayed the clinic diet in writing. Nowhere on the printed consent form was there a query about prescribed medications. There were, however, two other crucial questions: (1) Were any modifications to the program necessary? In her reply, the doctor made no mention of the pharmaceutical cornucopia she was prescribing, noting only that her patient was allergic to penicillin. (2) Did the doctor wish to receive regular reports on her patient's progress and physical condition? This one went unanswered.

Accordingly, the clinic didn't inform Juliette's physician that she was having a tough time. She lost only two pounds in the first six weeks. But then she went into a yo-yo pattern, with sudden drops of six or seven pounds, followed by mysterious gains of roughly the same amounts. During this time, her oblivious doctor renewed her prescriptions time and time again, despite being told by the pharmacist that Juliette was depleting some of them too quickly.

Three weeks into her diet, although Juliette's blood pressure was purportedly normal, her uric acid was sky high. The doctor sent her to a specialist for tests but inexplicably didn't receive the results for nineteen days. She was concerned enough about the report to arrange a repeat test, yet raised no objection to it being scheduled a good six weeks after the original alarming reading. The results of this one reached the doctor's office while she was on vacation. And after she returned, she didn't get around to reading them for about two more weeks. Then, she testified, she tried without success to reach her patient by phone.

Just a few days later, Juliette would be dead.

What had the specialist's report said? That the drastically dieting patient's condition was not being helped, but actually exacerbated, by every medication her doctor kept represcribing. And that she should be taken off them immediately.

Meanwhile, Juliette's weight kept fluctuating. Her ankles were swollen and her face was gaunt and sagging. She was so weak she couldn't leave the hotel room on a family visit to the Quebec Winter Carnival. She fainted three nights before her death, but didn't tell anyone except her mild-mannered husband, who obeyed her request to keep quiet about it. She was, however, so dizzy that she made a rare complaint on one of her last visits to the clinic. So the nurses, who were still recording reasonable blood pressure readings, allowed her the minuscule modification of adding a quarter-teaspoon of salt to her diet to slow down fluid loss.

But it was too little and too late. On her way home from work one day that spring, less than four months after starting what she had ironically vowed would be her last diet, Juliette stopped off at the Weight Loss Clinic. She walked across the lobby, crumpled to the floor, and died.

Nobody to Blame

The autopsy failed to reveal a specific cause of death, but two expert inquest witnesses testified that it was almost certainly arrhythmia (irregular heartbeats). This dangerous condition is well known to be brought on by the loss of potassium associated with diuretics, and it has also been linked with the other medications Juliette had been taking for years.

When all the testimony was complete, the coroner sent the jury off to deliberate, reminding them that their duty was not to ascribe blame to anyone but, rather, to come up with recommendations for preventing similar calamities in the future. Two hours later, they came back with a dozen eminently sensible suggestions. Then the inquest was over.

But not for me. I kept thinking that *somebody* must be to blame. The doctor, for her bumbling incompetence. The pharmacist, for not finding a way to override the doctor's okay on overlapping prescriptions. The Weight Loss Clinic, for taking such a big chunk of Juliette's money and then not only failing to help her lose weight but letting her wither in front of their eyes.

But what about Juliette? Was she actually responsible for killing herself? Could she possibly have been courting disaster subconsciously, or even deliberately, as a form of punishing herself—just as I had by visiting the circus Fat Lady? Could her reckless behavior really have sprung from simple ignorance of pharmaceutical dangers? Or was this to have been the ultimate atonement for the "sin" a lifetime of hearing antifat propaganda had convinced her she'd committed?

She certainly hadn't said anything of the kind, judging by what I heard at the inquest. But there had been a lot of testimony suggesting that she rarely spoke about her physical problems at all, and I knew this was a trait she shared with many obese people. We have the feeling that we aren't entitled to complain. Actually, we are loath to speak of our bodies at all, hoping that if we don't, we may escape the disgust that accompanies the inevitable attribution of gluttony.

Juliette left no conclusive evidence to prove this, but logic and informed intuition convinced me that what she probably did during the last few weeks of her life was panic about her fast-approaching deadline. Her yo-yo weight levels had to have been caused by binge-ing—probably in a desperate grab for energy to get through the day—followed by doubling, or possibly even tripling, her diuretics so that water loss would make her feel that she was succeeding. If my theory is correct, the wonder is that she survived as long as she did.

Juliette never made it to her deadline, but mine was getting closer and closer. In a fog of outrage, exhaustion, and fear, I wrote her story. My editors liked it, but they requested a rewrite. They told me to conceal the fact that my own life was wracked by the same obsession that killed Juliette. After raising a feeble objection, I ended up agreeing that doing so would enhance the appearance of pristine journalistic objectivity.

But I knew even then that I had really capitulated because I felt mortified. I had forced myself to "bleed onto the page" (to use a writer's term) because it was impossible to interview Juliette, and her family could tell me little because they never understood what drove her to a lifetime of dieting. But I was positive I knew that what put her in mortal danger was the agony of obsessively pursu-ing a goal you never manage to reach. And I had said so in the only way I could.

Yet when talented wordsmiths didn't consider my own ordeal appropriate to the story, I thought *I* must be the one who wasn't see-ing straight. It wasn't until years later, when I stopped doubting my own judgment, that I realized my editors had simply been embar-rassed by my candor. And that what really prompted the bowdleriza-tion was squeamishness about my admitting to being one of society's untouchables. "Obese" just wasn't a dignified status for smart people like us.

Nevertheless, I was initially quite proud of the story. I enjoyed a fair amount of praise, and people said it was a powerful piece. None of us realized that I had missed the most important element of all. Yes, I captured the *how* in exhaustive detail. But I never even speculated as to *why* Juliette was so driven, for so long, to become thin. The closest I came was a paragraph that was never published:

> I know, as she knew, the demons that drive a young girl, a teenager, and a young adult to deny herself a moment's peace about her appearance (which she's been brainwashed into interpreting as her worth). But Juliette had a couple of decades on me, as well as an adoring husband and loving offspring. It terrifies me to contemplate her example: another twenty years of anguish and then, finally, failure to conquer either the flesh or the obsession.

Fifteen of the twenty years that separated Juliette and me have now passed. As it turned out, I learned no more from her than I did from looking at the Fat Lady. I had written in horrified tones about Juliette's self-imposed privations, but continued inflicting them (all but the drugs) on myself. I had condemned weight loss surgery as "brutal enough to make a medieval torturer cringe," but had my stomach stapled just three years later. And then, when nothing worked and I remained fat no matter what I did, I spent the next decade slowly sinking into isolation and hopelessness. Then, literally when I least expected it, my redemption found me. I began doing research for this book and discovered what was missing from the story about the woman who dropped dead at the weight loss center.

The inquest jury hadn't been allowed to assign blame, and the closest I'd come was to implicitly fault Juliette herself for being fatally obsessed. After which I unconsciously imitated her example for a decade and a half, ultimately escaping to the bitter haven of anonymity, and remaining mired in the same obsession. All the while, I assumed that I had only myself to blame.

But I couldn't have been more wrong. Nor could Juliette. The truth is, we were exactly like hopeless laboratory rats. There was no way out of the maze we'd been duped and coerced into entering. We were *supposed* to fail, and then to keep on failing. That's how the billion-dollar brainwash works. It's the only way millions of people can be robbed of billions of dollars, year after futile year. Juliette just did it all a little too well.

Secret Casualties of a Secret War

I have retold Juliette Christie's tragic story here because she epito-
mizes the hundreds—possibly even thousands—of other women
throughout North America who are virtually murdered by antifat
forces every year. A wild exaggeration? I'm afraid not. When you add
in those who die from weight loss surgery, plus those whose lives are
sacrificed to anorexia and bulimia, plus the many who perish because
they try to control their weight by smoking, we may be talking about
tens of thousands.

But guess what? Nobody's keeping score. We never hear the names
of the casualties in what amounts to a secret war. We aren't even told
that they die, let alone why. And if we do happen to find out, blame
is never assigned to anything but, at most, foolish, inexplicable vanity.
Why in the world do women do these things to themselves? Tsk, tsk.
What a shame.

Obliviousness and flat-out indifference, even on the part of national
authorities whose duty is to safeguard public health, made trying to
ferret out the mortality rate attributable to weight loss efforts the most
frustrating part of the research for this book. Ultimately failing to
dredge up irrefutable proof about the grisly toll the billion-dollar
brainwash is exacting has been a bitter disappointment for me.

I had begun my research confidently enough, with the standard
writer's technique of checking periodical indices and electronic databanks to see what facts other journalists had come up with, and to find
clues about relevant authorities to interview. But none of the many
"keywords" and topic combinations I tried paid off. There was *nothing*
to be found about deaths resulting from drastic diets, fasts, bariatric
surgery, contributing chemical abuse (such as Juliette's), or even eating disorders.

I moved on to major newspapers. *Nothing*—except multiple articles
about the risks of obesity, sprinkled with many sky-is-falling quotes
from profitmongers themselves, whose endorsement of various reducing schemes should be considered conflicts of interest, instead of obediently reported as genuine news.

I saved what I thought would be a research treasure trove for last:
the health databanks. Surely, I thought, abundant attention must have

been paid to the fatal consequences connected with practices that millions of people have engaged in on a daily basis for decades. But I was astounded to be proven wrong.

So I decided to play the only trump card I had. I punched into the library computer the one victim's name I knew for sure: singer Karen Carpenter, the most famous casualty to date of the weight obsession epidemic. People all over the world knew her music and were stunned when she died of anorexia in 1983 at the age of thirty-two. Her tragedy prompted the hundreds of news stories it deserved, and shocked the public into focusing on a disease few had previously known about. But—just a decade after her death—she has practically become a missing person. There are hardly any references to Carpenter in the databanks for the 1990s.

Discovering this sinister blank was so upsetting that I began to wonder if fatalities had somehow been deliberately "disappeared." But even I don't really think that's it. After striking out—despite thorough checking with the American Medical Association, the National Institutes of Health, the Centers for Disease Control and Prevention, the National Center for Health Statistics, the American College of Surgery, the American Society of Bariatric Physicians, the American Society of Bariatric Surgery, the National Library of Medicine, and the American Hospital Association, among other organizations—I came up with more plausible answers.

One: The inescapable prothinness message preached on behalf of the billion-dollar brainwash drowns out the few voices that question or contradict it, resulting in a "dumbing down" of not only the general population, but most health authorities as well.

Two: "Hush money" is another crucial reason why weight-loss-related deaths aren't hitting the headlines. This theory isn't just mine, it was also the conclusion of researchers at the National Institutes of Health's Obesity Research Center in New York, who reviewed private records regarding a number of abandoned lawsuits. They reported in a recent issue of the *Healthy Weight Journal*—which, to my knowledge, is the only publication even trying to keep track of the mortality rate in this context—that weight-loss-related fatalities, including "Sudden Death Syndrome," are actually common. But whenever survivors sue for wrongful death, defendants generally try to settle out of court, on condition that the plaintiffs keep their mouths shut forever.

Three: The failure to even count how many people are being sacrificed in the name of thinness is systemic—merely one more cruel, disrespectful disservice done to those whose legitimate membership in the human race has been all but canceled by antifat profiteers.

There's a major story to be told here, with the possibility of uncovering thousands of secret deaths, plus massive custodial oversight, and possibly even payoffs somewhere along the line. This makes the situation juicy enough to tempt a tabloid. But it will surely take a skilled investigative journalist from the mainstream media to penetrate the dead end that defeated me—namely, that mortality statistics of all kinds are tabulated and analyzed according to data collected from death certificates. And there is no such cause-of-death category as "excessive reducing," let alone "waif syndrome"— the appropriate name if a sorely needed new category of such fatalities is ever instituted.

What I Did Uncover

The little known facts that prodigious digging *did* reveal are shocking. Examples:

- At least fifty-eight deaths have been blamed on liquid-protein diets (such as Oprah and I endured) since their introduction in the 1970s. Yet they're still in use, and recently became available without doctors' prescriptions.
- Diet pills containing the now-famous "fen-phen" combination were blamed for between twenty and forty deaths per year in France, and at least seventy-eight incurable cases of a lung disease called primary pulmonary hypertension (PPH), before their restriction in that country in 1995. Yet the same combination of fenfluramine and dexfenfluramine is enjoying spectacular popularity here, especially since the FDA's controversial 1996 approval of a form called Redux—which was issued despite a study published in the *New England Journal of Medicine* charging that using fen-phen for longer than three months increases the risk of PPH by about 3,000 percent.

• Thirty heart attack deaths were attributed to the vastly popular Cambridge Diet—an insufficiently nutritious meal replacement powder—before the FDA finally banned it.

• Two dozen deaths have resulted from herbal diet potions bearing such names as Mini Thin, Diet Max, Excel Diet, Lacey LeBeau Super Dieter's Tea, and Thermogen Herbal Tea, thanks to their major active ingredient—ephedrine—which can speed up heart rates, elevate blood pressure, precipitate strokes, and thus prove fatal. Yet the FDA's regulatory hands are tied because these are technically not food products.

• Nine of the first women who underwent liposuction died soon afterward in France. Nevertheless, the procedure was approved for use in North America and quickly became the most frequently performed of all cosmetic surgeries. Result: At least twenty deaths during its first six years here, according to a congressional subcommittee, and authorities evidently suspect that liposuction is currently producing many more deaths.

• General suicide rates among people with "weight problems" remain unknown. But a report in the *American Journal of Psychiatry* estimated that weight-loss-surgery patients kill themselves at a significantly higher rate than those who are morbidly obese* but do not choose to have operations.

Certainly, no one in the medical community is likely to conclude that extreme obesity is good for anyone's health. But does being overweight to a lesser degree automatically mean an early death sentence, as we're being led to believe? The answer, acccording to a growing number of authorities, is no.

A recent report by the Institute of Medicine, for instance, concluded that the assumption simply does not stand up to the facts—which are, basically, that during the past few decades, as Americans grew fatter, fewer actually died from the culprits most commonly linked to obesity. In other words, the incidence of cardiac disease, high blood pressure, and high cholesterol has declined, rather than risen.

---

*Weighing 100 pounds more than what's currently considered to be proportionally average.

The truth is that drastic reducing methods, especially when their repetition produces yo-yo weight levels, can often be more dangerous than being moderately heavy. So can being significantly underweight, as opposed to steadily maintaining a somewhat higher weight level. Put even more succinctly by epidemiologist Steven N. Blair, "One of the fundamental tenets of the weight loss industry is if you get people to eat less, they'll lose weight . . . and be better off." But, as he reported to a 1994 American Heart Association meeting, "there is no evidence to support either [contention]."

Blair backed up what is still considered a controversial statement by citing the results of an important study (inexplicably limited to males, despite the fact that an estimated 90 percent of dieters are female). It determined that, among chronic dieters, as compared with overweight subjects who weren't in the habit of dieting, heart disease was more than twice as prevalent, hypertension was 15 percent more common, and diabetes occurred five times more often.

As for those who do die because of weight loss attempts, the most typical examples, according to a variety of medical professionals, are women whose basic health starts out as good. Why do they end up dead? Most commonly, because of total fasting, severely restricted regimens (usually below 600 calories), weight loss surgery, or the tricky refeeding periods that routinely follow fasting and surgery.

The direct causes of these deaths are frequently arrhythmia; electrolyte abnormalities; nutritional inadequacy, including a lack of minerals such as potassium, magnesium, and copper; and grossly reduced heart weight. Pre- and postoperative stress belong on this list as well, according to Dr. Janis Fisler, of UCLA's cardiology division. Her conclusion, arrived at after investigating dieting deaths for the past decade, is based in part on the fact that bariatric surgery patients often suffer such acute anxiety that even something as innocuous as a loud noise can trigger fatal arrhythmia.

A Silent Epidemic of Eating Disorders

Then there are the "formal" eating disorders of anorexia and bulimia, about which I had no trouble getting reliable statistics. They're even grimmer than I had supposed. The total number of American females with eating disorders has now topped 11 million, according to the National Association of Anorexia Nervosa and Associated Disorders. And the mortality rate is believed to be between 10 and 15 percent.

To put this in some sort of perspective—but without meaning to minimize the catastrophe of AIDS—there are 50 times more women on this continent who suffer from eating disorders than there are female HIV/AIDS patients. But no colored ribbons are worn to call attention to, or express compassion for, those who have been felled, mostly in secret, by the illogical edict that all women must be thin.

When they don't die, at least 80 percent of anorexics and bulimics suffer multiple relapses before being cured. And both types of eating disorder can be accompanied by so many side effects that their victims often become physically and psychologically incapacitated. These include hypothermia, dehydration, electrolyte imbalance, low blood pressure, abnormal heart rhythm, kidney failure, hiatal hernia, tooth erosion (from frequent exposure to stomach acid), esophageal damage, infertility, osteoporosis, and depression.

Bulimia is considered even less reversible than anorexia, mostly because its physical effects are less obvious and allow those affected to hide their behavior more successfully than anorexics. Consequently, bulimia has been known to persist for decades, just as it did in Jane Fonda's case. While we were watching her smiling through her movies, she was forcing herself to throw up as many as twenty times a day.

How do these disasters get started? For many victims, the answer to that key question is clear. What starts out as a quick crash diet to lose a modest amount of weight—say, just enough to look like a favorite fashion model—simply spirals out of control.

Actresses, whose appearance is, regrettably, still their number one career qualification, are particularly vulnerable. Among those whose eating disorders have become public knowledge, in addition to Fonda, are Sally Field, Lynn Redgrave, Sandra Dee, Ally Sheedy, Tracey Gold, and Janine Turner. Other kinds of performers are also at risk, and the known casualty list includes comedian Joan Rivers, dancers Paula Abdul and Gelsey Kirkland, and singer Cherry Boone (daughter of Pat Boone).

Athletes, especially female, also frequently become trapped in eating disorders. Olympic gymnast Christy Henrich, for example, dropped to just 47 pounds before she died of anorexia in 1994, and her death was widely reported. Yet much of the media coverage was as obtuse as that of *Allure* magazine, which pointedly entitled an excellent article on Henrich "Starved to Death," yet featured "superwaif" Kate Moss on the cover of that edition, and nothing but ultra-thin models throughout it.

No internationally famous women, besides Carpenter and Henrich, have so far lost their lives because they wanted to be thin—at least not according to news reports. In reality, at least two such senseless deaths have occurred. But, in both instances, what we heard were not the pertinent facts but, rather, moronic jokes about what gluttons the deceased dieters must have been.

One of these women was Christina Onassis, the former stepdaughter of Jacqueline Kennedy Onassis, and the sole surviving heir to the Greek shipping empire of her father, Aristotle Onassis. Her 1988 death, at age thirty-eight, was chalked up to (and may indeed have been precipitated by) a drug overdose. But the fact is, Onassis had jeopardized her health for decades by embarking on reckless weight loss regimens, trying in vain to transform her genetic chunkiness into the willowy dimensions demanded of the glamorous jet-setters who populated her world.

The second celebrated casualty was Mama Cass Elliot, the most popular member of one of the top singing groups in America during the mid-1960s, the Mamas and the Papas. Her 1974 death in London at the age of thirty-three provoked an onslaught of cruel quips. The worst of them sprang from a report out of Los Angeles that Elliot had choked to death while eating a ham sandwich. The anonymous conjecture was soon proven false by the results of an autopsy which revealed a fatal heart attack to be the cause of death. Yet the sick joke instantly rocketed around the world and quickly entered popular folklore. After all, what could possibly be a funnier or more fitting demise for a Fat Chick? Live by the sandwich, die by the sandwich.

Ignored during the callous chuckle-fest that has lasted for twenty-three years have been Elliot's desperate and repeated attempts to reduce her famously rotund body to what she called "the promised land of 110 pounds." Before these efforts robbed her of her life, they had already cost her the stellar solo career to which she had been headed.

Elliot had left the Mamas and the Papas at the height of the quartet's success. Her sassy style and soaring mezzo-soprano voice had attracted legions of fans and reams of fulsome praise that was epitomized later by an obituary in the *New York Times* calling her "proof that one didn't have to be beautiful or thin to be successful and idolized."* But the admiration that many another large woman would practically kill for couldn't budge Elliot's obsession with slimming down. Nor could widespread reports that she had become a breakthrough role model. "Wherever the group appeared," said a contemporary *Esquire* article, "little fat girls would seek Cass out, ask her advice on their careers, and sit at her feet talking about life. . . . What Streisand did for Jewish girls in Brooklyn, [she] was doing for fat girls everywhere. The diet-food people . . . hated her the way nose surgeons are said to hate Streisand."

No matter. Elliot had decided that her new career must, and would, have a newly sculpted body. Sure enough, she dropped from 285 to 175 pounds in less than a year's time, according to an article she wrote for *Ladies' Home Journal* in 1969. What did it take? Fasting, without medical supervision, for nine grueling months, eating nothing between Mondays and Thursdays, and only a single evening meal of steak and a green vegetable between Fridays and Sundays. How did this horrendous program affect the singer? In her own words, it gave her "acute tonsillitis, hemorrhaging vocal cords, mononucleosis, and a dangerous case of hepatitis."

Before she had a chance to begin restoring her health, Elliot flew to Las Vegas to make her debut. Glittering Caesar's Palace was packed with celebrities and reporters, all confident they were about to see the launching of a superstar. Instead, they witnessed a humiliating debacle. The singer's energy was nil, her focus and timing were off, and, according to one reviewer, her "normally lithe voice was reduced to a crusty whisper." Elliot's engagement at Caesar's was canceled on the

---

*Need I point out that this remark dates from before the billion-dollar brainwash got into full swing?

spot, and she left Las Vegas, not on a jet, but in an ambulance. She later said that she had "lost my health—and more than a quarter of a million dollars in earnings." During the last five years of her life, Mama Cass struggled mightily to rebuild her career and to slim her body down to the improbable ideal she still cherished. She didn't succeed in either quest. And then, as if all this weren't sad enough, her memory was defiled by cruel jokes that have lasted for more than two decades.

How can I be certain that Onassis and Elliot died as a direct consequence of their obsession with being thin? I can't. And no one else seems to have been interested in investigating this possibility. But when I correlated the mortal risks described above with the known recklessness of these women's reducing efforts, I believe I discovered the truth. Would knowing why Onassis and Elliot really died have had a "miner's canary" effect and thus mitigated the disastrous situation created by the billion-dollar brainwash? It's hard to say. But I, for one, wish I had known all these years—instead of hearing nothing but heartless humor based, especially in the case of Mama Cass, on the assumption that these Fat Chicks got what they deserved.

Our Sisters' Keepers

No one was able to talk Juliette Christie out of a lifetime of dieting. Her husband testified at her inquest that he'd often tried to reassure her that he "liked her just as she was." And her daughter said she'd tried many times to help Juliette accept the fact that "some people are just meant to be big." But neither their patient persuasion nor their abiding love was powerful enough to undo the psychological damage done by the billion-dollar brainwash. In the end, even the people who loved Juliette best were unable to save her life.

But at least they tried. Many of us can't summon up the right words, or the courage to say them, when people we care about seem to be drifting into danger because of their obsession with being thin. I must count myself among this group of chicken-hearts.

One of my dearest friends, whose adult weight stabilized at an average level for many years (after some juvenile chubbiness), suddenly began losing weight a few years ago. Discreet queries elicited only the information that she had discovered fitness training. When I saw her again recently after an interval of three years, her body had dwindled down to what seemed like shocking thinness. Yet I somehow couldn't find the words to ask her point-blank how it happened. In every other way, she was the same wise, intensely funny, acutely aware woman I'd known for more than fifteen years. We spent only a few hours together during a reunion, so I found it easy to rationalize not bringing the subject up. But even though we're separated again, I certainly know her phone number and address, and could tell her about my concern. So why haven't I?

The closest I can come to answering is to remind myself that I've always had a hands-off policy, unless someone specifically asks for advice. My own body has been criticized so cruelly throughout my life that I'm reluctant to venture even a gentle cavil about someone else's. Feeble excuses? Definitely. But they're all I've got. So I'm hoping that my beloved friend will recognize herself when she reads this and volunteer answers to the questions I've been too cowardly to ask. And that this failure to act, on the part of someone who knows all too well what's at stake, will serve as a galvanizing influence on others whose silence may be imperiling their loved ones.

Bottom Line

Thanks to three decades of incessant, inescapable indoctrination by the multifaceted factions I call the billion-dollar brainwash, millions of Americans deprive and exhaust themselves every day of the year, trying to become unrealistically thin. At least 90 percent are women whose lives are, at best, restricted and, at worst, poisoned by the implacable pressure to do so. In my view, this should automatically make the obsession with weight loss, and the dangerous behavior it encourages, a top priority with medical and public-health officials, the news media, and, especially, women's organizations and publications.

But—as demonstrated by my fruitless search for even something as fundamental as the total number of people who die every year just from trying to lose weight—apparently no one in a position of authority sees the situation in this light. A highly placed associate at the Centers for Disease Control and Prevention told me, off the record, that

he seriously doubted *anyone* would be able to track the mortality rate.
Did that concern him? I asked. "Not particularly," he replied, in a
matter-of-fact tone.

I was so flummoxed that anyone dedicated to controlling major diseases would express such indifference—when the annual death toll
may well be in the thousands—that I didn't know what to say. So I just
thanked him for his time and hung up the phone.

Then I went for a long walk amidst tumbling autumn leaves. Their
cascading colors reminded me of the same season years ago, when I
was trying so desperately to make a third of my body vanish. And
when I was so afraid that I, too, would become one of the casualties
no one wants to talk about.

I thought some more about Juliette. I never got to meet her, yet I
feel as though I did. It's probably because I *am* her in so many ways.
We struggled with an identical obsession for an identical length of
time. We were both dupes of the same despicable profiteers. And both
of us starved, physically and psychologically, for years and years, subsisting on little more than hope and magazine dreams.

The only essential difference between Juliette and me is that she
can never awaken from the brainwashing. She died, just like Karen
Carpenter, Christy Henrich, Christina Onassis, and Mama Cass Elliot,
and untold numbers of other women whose names we may never
know. But I lived. And I finally learned that beauty, especially the
phony, tawdry, supremely superficial version we've been force-fed for
decades, is not worth dying for.

12

Belly-Up?

Glaring evidence of the billion-dollar brainwash and its terrible toll surrounds us—yet it remains one of our culture's dirtiest little secrets. No one wants to tell the truth about it or even admit it exists. There's just too much money to be made by telling the Big Lies that make us spend so obsessively.

But the reality is that the No Fat Chicks era is repeating the self-defeating scenario Betty Friedan revealed in 1963, when she wrote *The Feminine Mystique*. Her book detailed how what was won during the struggle for female suffrage was forgotten during the Depression and the Second World War and was squandered thereafter. But, women assured one another at the peak of modern feminist activity, such a profound loss couldn't possibly happen again now that our eyes are open.

It *is* happening again. And this time the losses aren't the result of unavoidable historic calamities. This time the dispossession is deliberate, and the technique of crushing women's core self-respect has resulted in an undermining of the momentous social and economic gains we have made during the past three decades. We have never had more freedom of choice and opportunity; but we have never felt worse about our bodies. So bad, in fact, that many of us would willingly accept early death in return for being thin.

Yet the most brilliant technique of the antifat profiteers is hiding their puppet strings so effectively that women honestly believe they are thinking for themselves and freely making their own choices about how they want to look and behave. Thus, some of those I interviewed for this book responded with blank confusion. Others indignantly denied that they're being forced, or even duped, into denying their appetites and driving themselves through busy days in a perpetual state of semi-starvation. Still others insisted that I'm overcomplicating the situation. Women have always wanted to look "nice," they said. That's all there is to it. And the fact that, at this particular point in time, "nice" happens to mean "thin," which happens to require prodigious expense and effort, just . . . sort of happened.

That the logical cause-and-effect continuum has escaped these people shouldn't be too surprising. It also seems to be as dead as a dodo in most other cultural contexts. When the occasional lonely voice does try to point out how the sky is falling upon us, the warnings simply waft in one collective ear and out the other. Amid dogged denial of even fundamentally inimical influences on our lives, it's obviously been a snap to smudge the connection between the high-pressure sales techniques of the billion-dollar brainwash and

- the epidemic of obesity;
- the spiraling scourge of eating disorders;
- the escalating incidence of clinical depression in the female population;
- the thousands of women who spend millions of dollars to have chunks of their own flesh lopped off, sucked out, or stapled shut;
- the millions more who "voluntarily" restrict their food intake to the point of courting malnutrition, exhaustion, and other medical calamities;
- and the many, many more who overexercise; smoke; abuse laxatives, diuretics, and amphetamines; pop dangerous diet drugs as if they were vitamins; and eschew birth control pills for the sake of being slender.

Even when a woman actually drops dead at a weight loss center, we're so well indoctrinated that we ignore the glaring object lesson and chalk it up to simple vanity. Any fool knows the dead woman only had herself to blame for getting fat in the first place.

Any fool? Exactly. That's what the antifat profiteers have made of us in the three decades since Twiggy let the genie of avarice out of the bottle by being catapulted into the beauty equation thanks to the social and demographic elements *Vogue*'s Diana Vreeland dubbed a "youthquake." She also remarked that "Twiggy couldn't have arrived at any other time. It's just as though this little old egg had been lying on the ground, and suddenly, on the right day, it hatched."

Vreeland's imagery is interesting viewed in retrospect. In fact, it's arguably less an egg than a modern equivalent of Pandora's box. For inside it was something that gradually metamorphosed from an emaciated teenager into an *idea* that was powerful enough to shift public opinion, perception, prejudice, and appetites through 180 degrees. The idea was, of course, that the strong, fertile, womanly sized women who've been favored throughout history, by nature, men, and artists, would henceforth be deemed a caste of untouchables.

During the next three decades, a host of virtual incubators saw to it that every woman who didn't, couldn't, or (in increasingly rare instances) wouldn't knuckle under to the Eleventh Commandment—Thou shalt not be fat—was punished and penalized so severely that she became a virtual teaching aid to reinforce the lesson among her slimmer sisters.

Fat Chicks—which is how *every* unslender woman was regarded by the time the profitable propaganda hit high gear—were not only stigmatized, stereotyped, and lied about in all the vehicles of popular culture, but hobbled by orchestrated intolerance at every turn. The process included being prevented from receiving decent health care, deprived of rewarding employment opportunities, robbed of both romantic relationships and the children that might have resulted from them, denied the social and professional advantage of dressing appropriately, lured into mortal danger, and generally laughed right out of their status as normal human beings.

All the while, Fat Chicks were taught to blame themselves for their misery. Every message carried by every medium that inundated their lives reinforced this reprehensible "logic." In time, they internalized the blame so thoroughly that it paralyzed both their common sense and their instinct for self-preservation. So they struggled to conform with what was expected of them, and spent every cent they could possibly spare. But nothing worked and they just grew fatter. That, of course, was also regarded as their fault.

Trying to explain that they actually ate less, not more, than many other women, or that science has now proven it's incessant dieting that keeps people fat, was just as pointless as trying to fight back. Nobody listened. So Fat Chicks thought in their darkest moments that maybe they really were guilty of the horrendous crime everyone had convicted them of. And if that were true, then all the punishment made sense because they deserved it.

Thus did the despicable hoax I call the billion-dollar brainwash poison my life decade after wasted decade, just as it still threatens the health and compromises the happiness of millions of other women and girls who are deliberately taught to hate their bodies. *Whatever* our weight, we are flimflammed into forgetting that nature creates us in a rich variety of shapes and sizes—and into believing that anyone who cannot permanently clone the physique of the thinnest 5 percent of the female population is a contemptible, unlovable failure.

The futility and absurdity of trying to accomplish this senseless feat should have been obvious all along. In fact, women might just as easily have been told they all had to be six feet tall, and that to achieve this, they'd have to get along on three hours' sleep a night and ski at least an hour every day—all of which could ostensibly be accomplished by buying products to "help" them do so. But if greedy marketers had tried something *that* extreme, we would surely have seen through their ludicrous ploy, laughed uproariously, and told them to take a hike.

Yet such is the power of an equally unachievable edict that we've been coerced into everlasting pursuit of something just as unrealistic. And that means we're spending a fortune that's now fattening up assorted American weight loss profiteers by more than $50 billion a year.

Luring women onward, like the ultimate carrot, is the fairy tale of living happily ever after; while behind them, the whip of antifat prejudice cracks ever louder. Both carrot and whip are supplied in saturation quantities by the magazines, books, television shows, movies, videos, newspapers, and billboards that relentlessly teach us to pursue happiness, love, and self-esteem by shopping. What are we taught to buy? Whatever the marketers who pay the media to brainwash us wish to sell.

Granted, this modus operandi also applies to innumerable other commodities and is actually a rudimentary blueprint for any market-driven economy. But there's a crucial difference between hoodwinking someone into thinking that Brand X shampoo will make her the belle of the ball and browbeating her into believing that life isn't worth living unless she stays thin.

The Orwellian No Fat Chicks rule is inescapable. And like other evil campaigns that have swayed entire societies, it warps our perspective so severely that we use its message as a weapon against ourselves, each other, and every new generation. No female is safe from its corrosive influence—not a superstar entertainer, a wealthy heiress, a popular princess, a history-making prime minister, an obscure grandmother, or a bewildered schoolgirl.

Result: Millions of lives are being sacrificed psychologically, and the untold mortality rate may well number in the thousands. Like puppets dangling helplessly on invisible strings, we think what the antifat profiteers want us to think. We do what they want us to do. And we buy what they want us to buy.

And Yet . . .

At the risk of contradicting my own conclusions, I must now declare my belief that the beginning of the end of the brutal No Fat Chicks era is gradually coming into view. Why? Chiefly because of the demographic clout of the baby boomers. The antifat propagandists were always right about one thing: Money talks. The whole phenomenon couldn't have happened in the first place if there hadn't been a lot of cash jingling in the jeans of the 78 million American teenagers whom they conned into assuming that all women could, and should, look like Twiggy in perpetuity. Those same boomers are a lot older now. But they've still got "attitude" and they're still the sector with the most buying power.

A lot of marketers forgot that. Actually, what they forgot is that people age as time goes by, and kept assuming that focusing on the youth market—which had paid off so magnificently in the past—would be a surefire formula forever. Reality check: In the late 1990s, an American will turn fifty every 7.5 seconds. The trend will continue for seventeen years, and all the while, about 80 percent of these boomers will naturally "plump up" rather than "skinny down." In addition, many of these people are parents who are becoming more and more outraged at how the thinness obsession is ravaging the safety and happiness of their daughters. And, as many authorities have pointed out, every time the boomers say "gimme," sooner or later, they get what they want.

Small wonder, then, that there are scattered reports to the effect that the number of chronic American dieters has dropped during the past half-dozen years. A recent poll showed that the number of people who think "overweight" automatically means "unattractive" has also dipped. Another found that 65 percent of female respondents said they'd rather win a Pulitzer Prize than be Miss America. And several surveys have shown that, for the first time in more than a decade, neither women nor men are automatically making dieting their number one annual New Year's resolution.

The most prescient marketers have taken note of this trend and are beginning to respond in ways that simultaneously serve consumers and their own bottom lines—which is, after all, how capitalism is *supposed* to work. Most visible, of course, are the makers of low- and no-fat food products, the best of which are a boon for reasonable weight control. The year 1995 saw no fewer than 1,900 new entries into this arena.

A few companies are going even further, and deserve recognition and encouragement. Frito Lay, for example, is currently running hilarious ads featuring slender supermodels plus Miss Piggy feasting on, and bespeckled by, its baked potato crisps. The most admirable effort I am aware of is an advertising campaign for Kellogg's Special K cereal that began appearing in women's magazines in the fall of 1996. The most hard-hitting of these full-page ads shows a near-skeletal woman in a bikini beside copy reading, "If this is beauty, there's something wrong with the eye of the beholder." Another depicts a man with a huge belly overhanging his bathing trunks and a slender woman in her skivvies. The caption: "Ironically, she's the one who's worried about her weight." The most pointed among these ads features a portly, balding, middle-aged man garbed in typical women's haute couture clothes beside copy reading "If only designers had to live up to the same standards they've set for us."

Also encouraging is the fact that fashion designer Calvin Klein—the leading purveyor of advertising celebrating waif-sized women, young-

younger-youngest models, and nude-nuder-nudest photos*—backed down for the first time ever in the summer of 1995 and withdrew a multimillion-dollar ad campaign. Previously, he had only seemed flattered when his cheesy ads provoked outrage. But when a chorus of assorted complainants shouted that his latest sleazy photos had gone too far, Klein actually listened. Which means that, because he is arguably the primary trendsetter, the concept of responsibility is being reintroduced into fashion and advertising.

Proof of this proposition startled many an observer in Milan during fashion shows the following year, when designers organized a "Food is good" campaign, including a huge poster depicting a model avidly eating a bowl of pasta, and an "anti-anorexia party" featuring an array of delicious foods.

Another hopeful sign is the fact that artists, who are always the first to catch the whiff of a new wind when it blows in, have begun discovering the rich variety of creatively exploitable themes inherent in the scam of the century. There's oppression to be revealed, mortal secrets to be uncovered, heroic physical and psychological battles, and villains galore. So far, only a few writers, actors, directors, photographers, and television producers have "got it." But what they're creating is powerful. Examples:

- *Eating*,† one of writer/producer/director Henry Jaglom's trademark "pseudo-documentaries," effectively captures the anguished ambivalence of three dozen female friends who gather for a birthday party. As delectable food is passed from hand to hand, with almost no one partaking, each character reveals the lengths to which she has gone just to survive inside the straitjacket of slenderness. (My favorite line: "I'm looking for a man who's as satisfying as a baked potato." I laughed out loud, and the fact that most of the women at the movie did not made the point even stronger.)
- Before actress and TV talk show host Ricki Lake lost more than one hundred pounds, she starred in *Babycakes*, a Hollywood

*Klein once told *Vogue* "I've done everything I could do in a provocative sense without being arrested."

†For which the director auditioned 600 women, very few of whom did *not* profess eating disorders.

remake of a romantic German film called *Sugarbaby*. It is probably the only movie in cinematic history in which the male protagonist falls in love with—and leaves his slender wife for—an extremely large woman.

• English actress Minnie Driver was put on a "reverse diet" to gain twenty pounds to star in a charming film called *Circle of Friends*. The ugly-duckling-becomes-a-swan (without losing an ounce) plot involves the heroine's unexpected romance with the local "catch" (played by Chris O'Donnell), whose screen father utters a line of dialogue that must surely be a first: "There's a lot to be said," he tells his son, "for these big, soft girls." Meanwhile, several other actresses recently enhanced their film characters' credibility by gaining weight. They include Meryl Streep for *The Bridges of Madison County*; Toni Collette, who put on forty-two pounds to star in *Muriel's Wedding*, and "supermodel" Elle McPherson, who gained twenty pounds for *Sirens*. Of course, this trend actually began twenty-five years ago, when Twiggy deliberately "porked up" so she could launch an acting career.

• *Fat Chance: The Big Prejudice*, a National Film Board of Canada documentary that was the sleeper hit of the 1994 Toronto Film Festival, began with the premise that its star, a 370-pound social worker named Rick Zakowich, would attempt to lose half of his body weight, while cameras chronicled the odyssey. The premise seemed not only do-able but dramatically interesting, especially because the plan was to include abundant evidence of prejudice (such as a woman whose hatred of obesity is so intense that she refuses even to walk in a fat person's footsteps). But the film's plot took an unexpected turn when dieting and exercising proved to be not only futile, but despair inducing. As it turned out, it wasn't Zakowich's body but his attitude that was ultimately transformed for the better. And it was spending time with a variety of fight-back activists that accomplished the feat. Zakowich is at peace with himself at last and has become a size-acceptance crusader himself.

• Best of all in terms of reaching mass audiences, acclaimed director Steven Spielberg (*Schindler's List*, *E.T.*) is reportedly producing a feature film which is tentatively called *Body Image*. Screenwriter Andrea King says it's about "a beautiful, smart, sexy, fat woman."

- In theater, 270-pound actress Camryn Manheim wrote, staged, and performed a one-woman show called *Wake Up, I'm Fat* which was an off-Broadway hit in 1993. Manheim also did a tastefully shot nude scene in a movie called *The Road to Wellville* which *People* magazine said was so enthusiastically received that she was immediately cast in "not-fat roles" in two other films, and became a regular on a TV series called *The Practice*. *Blown Sideways Through Life* is another innovative one-woman stage show, written and performed by amply proportioned Claudia Shear, which was recently filmed and broadcast by PBS. In it, Shear declares that "to be fat is to be branded not merely unerotic, but un-American, unattractive, unaesthetic, undisciplined."

- As for novels, no one has yet topped Margaret Atwood's *Lady Oracle*, in which a young girl combats her mother's domination by deliberately eating her way to obesity. To comfort herself, the heroine indulges in delightful fantasies such as being a fat but beloved opera singer, with permission to "stand up there in front of everyone and shriek as loud as you could, about hatred and love and rage and despair, scream at the top of your lungs and have it come out music." But best-selling author Pat Conroy makes an effectively caustic jest in his most recent novel, *Beach Music*, to the effect that society won't be satisfied until bulimia is included in bridal vows. *The Dieter*, by Chicago-based novelist Susan Sussman, is another affecting look at the complicated psychological factors involved in carrying what society considers to be too much weight. Equally enlightening is Wally Lamb's *She's Come Undone*, whose obese protagonist struggles to survive a typical Fat Chick's life obstacles.

- In music, a new generation of female composers, led by country stars such as Shania Twain, Mary Chapin Carpenter, and Pam Tillis, is boldly demanding a better deal for women in dozens of new songs epitomized by a recent Michelle Wright hit, *New Kind of Love*. Its central message, repeated many times throughout the song, is that the world, and any man who wishes to befriend her, must accept her "just as I am."

- Among the visual artists who have begun reminding beholders that beauty doesn't always come in small packages is Lisa

Yuskavage, whose recent New York show of what she calls "big, fleshy, naked women," was praised in *Newsweek* as the "craftiest, funniest and . . . sexiest art around," and sold out in a single week. By the way, one of the hottest art tickets in years had droves of patrons rushing to Boston's Museum of Fine Arts recently to see the abundant damsels painted in the 1600s by Peter Paul Rubens.

- A few actresses are publicly bucking rampant emaciation in their profession, including Brett Butler, star of the hit TV series *Amazing Grace*, who recently told *Entertainment Weekly* that "I'm a big, healthy woman with sturdy feet."
- In a class by herself, and certainly the only person who can and does circulate subversive antibrainwash messages on a daily basis, in hundreds of newspapers, is cartoonist Cathy Guisewite. It's a rare day when her *Cathy* strip doesn't raise the consciousness of millions of readers with humorous jabs at a culture that's besotted with ridiculously unrealistic portrayals of skinny women.
- Television has also begun getting in on the act recently by broadcasting some excellent shows on such topics as dangerous weight loss surgery (*Prime Time Live*); the "fat and fit" movement (*20/20*); and the ludicrous amount of money people are spending to ride the diet roller coaster (CNN). The best eye-opener so far was a *Nick News* special called "The Body Trap" (Nickelodeon).

  Cohosted by Linda Ellerbee and Rosie O'Donnell, the program featured a lively discussion among youngsters about the role appearance plays in contemporary life. The most positive contribution came from some African American girls, whose matter-of-fact comments about size reflected their upbringing in the segment of our society that's the most realistic and relaxed about women's bodies. While the white girls on the show admitted that their standards regarding body image come from magazines, TV, and films, the black girls said their ideas were acquired from their own families.

Which brings me to what I consider to be the very best development of all in terms of putting an end to the No Fat Chicks era: the rocketing to stardom of Rosie O'Donnell. We've already discussed the tremendously powerful effect the careers of Oprah Winfrey and Roseanne have had on women who desperately needed positive role models. But I believe that riveting Rosie—whose sensationally popular talk show had the highest rated debut in TV history—may outdo them both as a catalyst for change. Why? To begin with, instead of being ashamed of her size, she is the poster child for self-acceptance. She's intensely funny, irresistably chummy, and obviously unconflicted about her weight, which, she says, ranges between 150 and 200 pounds. "I don't think that I'm less of a person because I'm bigger than some people, nor do I think I'm better when I'm thinner," she recently told *Ms.* magazine.

But the clincher to my theory that Rosie represents something brand new is that she's the only Rubenesque star who hasn't attracted a single fat joke. The closest anyone has come was a verbal blunder by singer Donny Osmond, which prompted disapproving headlines as far away as Israel, attracted scores of supportive letters for Rosie, and resulted in his doing penance on the show by begging Rosie's forgiveness, wearing a dog costume, and serenading her with *Puppy Love*. Similarly, after an ad for Scope mouthwash called O'Donnell "unkissable," the rival mouthwash company, Listerine, instantly offered to contribute $1,000 to children's charities for every time Rosie was kissed on her show. Celebrities stampeded to show their support, racking up more than $500,000 in donations. Trust me, nothing like this has *ever* happened to a Fat Chick before—at least not since Rubenesque Lillian Russell reigned supreme in the 1890s.

The More Things Change . . .

But these heartening harbingers add up to little more than a glimmer of hope. Overall, it's still mostly business as usual,* with the vast majority of people behaving as if an attitudinal about-face in this context is impossible. Even those who publicly deplore the pressure on women to be ultra-thin generally attribute it to inexplicable, intractable cultural forces. Nearly all commentators stop short of pos-

*Case in point: When *Woman's World* featured Rosie O'Donnell on its cover recently, it not only air-brushed her photo to look thinner, but positioned a headline reading "Miracle Diets in Your Future" over the top of her thighs.

ing—let alone answering—the obvious question this book addresses: Why did losing weight become an international obsession?

Most vocal and deliberate among these obfuscators, of course, are those who stand to lose big-time if millions of women snap out of the profitable trance and start living on their own terms, dreaming dreams of their own devising, and fulfilling them any way they see fit. But, both inside and outside the profiteering cartel, there's plenty of blame to spread around for perpetuating the No Fat Chicks era.

There are the celebrities, most notably Weight Watchers' Lynn Redgrave, Kathleen Sullivan, and most recently, Sarah Ferguson, the Duchess of York; Slim-Fast's Ann Jillian and Tommy Lasorda; and Jenny Craig's Cindy Williams. All assure us, ad nauseam, that permanent weight loss is a sure thing, and that it's only a phone call and a few dollars away. This has the effect of making millions of us feel like failures when we cannot duplicate the feats of the celebrities, who have the advantage of professional help, plus lavish encouragement and monetary rewards.

Even worse are those who become stars by losing weight and then turn into virulent antiobesity bigots. Rosemary Green, best-selling author of *Diary of a Fat Housewife*, calls herself "the last honest fat person in America" and regularly blabs on TV talk shows about the ugliness of obesity. Green actually wrote a letter to "Dear Abby" taking her to task for defending Fat Chicks ("Of course people are discriminated against because of their size! Do you want our next Miss America to weigh 237 pounds?"). And she littered her book with self-degrading, prejudice-reinforcing remarks such as "Did I oink out? Do dogs have fleas? Does chocolate have calories? Yes, yes, yes, and yes! Disgusting, horrible, despicable."

In a category all her own is recently retired, longtime *Cosmopolitan* editor Helen Gurley Brown. She was a hero in the early 1960s for almost single-handedly making women understand that the time we spent after growing up and before getting married didn't need to be an anxious, unrewarding race to get a ring on our fingers before being scorned as spinsters. But more recently, Brown, whose influence on the 16 million women throughout the world who read *Cosmo* was vast, became one of the worst "sizeist" bigots on the planet. Even in her autobiography, *The Late Show*, she makes such cracks as "Anybody who sits around rationalizing that she can eat what she wants to . . .

I'm afraid I think is an asshole" and "I feel superior to fat people, drinkers, drug users and real dummies."

Then there are government and legislative leaders, especially those whose mandate is protecting human and civil rights, who turn a blind eye to discrimination against the obese. As pioneering size-acceptance advocate Dr. Moe Lerner pointed out to me, "If you call a woman 'babe' or an African American 'boy,' you're in trouble with the law. But it's still socially and legally acceptable to call someone a 'big fat dope.' That's just [considered] fun."

There are the airlines, which often refuse to accommodate very large people, or automatically charge them for two seats and humiliate them in front of other passengers. A Los Angeles woman named Pam Hollowich, for example, recently sued Southwest Airlines because of a "terribly traumatic, degrading" incident she says involved a ticket agent pulling her out of line at the boarding gate and loudly demanding that she buy a second ticket on the spot.

There are the cinemas and other theaters which no longer routinely sprinkle in a few of the double-wide "sweetheart" seats that were commonplace thirty or forty years ago, yet refuse to allow large people to bring in their own chairs for use in the areas reserved for wheelchairs.

And there are the myriad publications that feature tobacco ads luring women and girls* into a potentially fatal trap by suggesting that smoking will keep them thin. Examples include ubiquitous full-page, full-color cigarette ads for Misty Lights, which repeat the operative term three times: "slim 'n sassy," "slim price, too," and "Slims" on the side of the pack. Similar tobacco advertisements (e.g., Capri's "the slimmest slim in town"), on which the industry spends $6 billion a year, are the life's blood of nearly all mass-circulation magazines and litter the landscape on blaring billboards. Recently, widespread anger about their cavalier attitude toward public health has prompted some cigarette marketers to substitute the transparent euphemism "light" for "slim."

Also in my "most despicable" category are the majority of the producers of TV shows aimed at children. These media bigwigs get rich from saturation advertising of food products that guarantee kids will

---

*Teenage girls are currently the fastest-growing cohort among all smokers, and represent the majority of the estimated three thousand American teenagers who start smoking every day of the year.

develop weight problems—thus manufacturing future customers for the billion-dollar brainwash. A recent report from the National Center for Health Statistics showed that obesity has more than doubled in the six-to-seventeen age group since the 1960s. Small wonder when, according to Yale University obesity researcher Kelly D. Brownell, "the average child sees 10,000 food commercials a year . . . 95 percent of which are for . . . sugared cereals, soft drinks, and fast food."

And another troubling aspect of entertainment aimed at children is the hypersexy images of the female characters in animated movies such as Disney's *Beauty and the Beast*, *Aladdin*, and *Pocahontas*, and cartoons like *Sailor Moon* and *The Power Rangers*. Anyone who claims to be mystified as to where little girls get the idea they have to be thin (and have large breasts), and how little boys develop their notion of female attractiveness, need look no further than these examples.

Then there are the educators who allow fat youngsters to be attacked and excluded throughout their childhood. And, later on in their academic lives, according to several studies, fat teenage girls are at least 33 percent less likely to be selected for top colleges than slimmer students with identical academic qualifications.

And last, but by no means least, in terms of cruelty to everyone who is noticeably fat, there is the general public, in far too substantial numbers. The legacy of antifat and antidiversity attitudes they bestow on their children results in overweight youngsters being the first to be taunted and the last to be chosen for sports and other activities. It continues with "just happening" to forget to invite overweight teenagers to parties. It rolls onward every time someone tells an antiobesity joke or laughs at one. And it ends up preventing wider-than-waif women from being seen for who they really are, punishing them for things they aren't, depriving them of many of their legal and human rights, and generally making their lives a living hell.

Although *No Fat Chicks* was a horrifying story to write, living through the era inside a Lillian Russell–size body was much worse. But when my research and analysis made me realize that the thinness edict was never really about weight at all, but simply about money, I made the joyful discovery that to see through the scam is to be liberated from its clutches.

The war with my body is finally over. I won.

And so can others, despite the overwhelming odds I'm attempting to expose. My fiercest wish is that this book will inspire women and girls, whatever their size, to repeat for themselves what simple knowledge empowered me to do: awaken from the obsession, open the door of a painful psychological prison, and step out free forever. If they do so in massive numbers, the billion-dollar brainwash will—to use an apt colloquialism—go belly-up.

Ending the No Fat Chicks Era

What can *you* do to guarantee that this happens? Plenty.

Start by really listening when little girls express their admiration for the grotesque body standard epitomized by the Barbie doll.* Listen to older girls bemoaning their imaginary fatness. Listen to your own friends complaining about those proverbially unbudgeable ten pounds. Listen to yourself whenever a glance in the mirror elicits an automatic reproach. Then realize that we've all been obediently mouthing lines from a script written by robbers.

The next time you flip through a women's magazine, really *see* the towering, expressionless, flat-hipped, exclusively young women with the disproportionately large breasts plopped on their chests like bizarre merit badges. Check out the pathetically bony shoulders, stringy arms, and emaciated legs of supermodels such as Claudia Schiffer as they lope along the fashion runways. When you watch television, count the number of hollow cheeks, protruding clavicles, and jutting hipbones among the actresses. Then think about whose interests—even beyond the antifat profiteers—are best served by keeping women so tiny and frail.

Whenever you're stuck in a checkout line, really look at the double-dealing magazine covers that hook us with headlines lecturing us about losing weight, and photos of delectable food that lead us into temptation—and then back to dieting.

---

*Incidentally, 90 percent of all American girls ages three to eleven own one or more Barbie dolls, which have been sold in the multimillions since 1959, and which, blown up to life size, would measure a preposterous 40-18-33, and have too little body fat for menstruation.

Realize that, like the slaves of yore, you have been sold to marketers by magazines and other popular media vehicles—and that you are paying for your complicity.

Watch for the next big "scientific" study bemoaning our "epidemic of obesity." And then figure out which giant conglomerate sponsored it just to soften up consumers for its next diet-product launch.

Connect the dots whenever you hear so-called experts, who are actually mouthpieces for these companies, loudly attacking every promising discovery of genetic causes, or possible cures, for obesity.

Ask yourself—or better yet, the media who repeat these dubious stories—why we don't see equivalent headlines about the devastating fallout from obsessive weight loss efforts, including a virtual epidemic of eating disorders.

Recognize that the attitude that attacks large people is actually the precise kind of social discrimination that has finally become unacceptable in every other context.

Think about how wonderful it would feel to know that you've dieted for the last time.

Get inspired by reading some of the revolutionary books I've quoted, as well as a welcome raft of new ones, including *Thin Is Just a Four-Letter Word*, by plus-size fitness instructor Dee Hakala, and *Well Rounded*, by plus-size model Catherine Lipponcott. All contain exhilarating words like these, from *When Women Stop Hating Their Bodies*: "Imagine this: You get up in the morning, turn on the TV and as you dress for work, you listen to the news being reported by an anchorwoman who wears a size 20. On the bus to work, you flip through your favorite magazine, which this month, miraculously, contains no ads that use women's bodies to sell products. During your coffee break, you enjoy the company of other women in your office, and not one of you, even for a moment, talks about dieting or weight."

Watch for evidence that the attitudinal tide is turning, and then tell everyone you can. Examples: Two women who are getting not just mad but even are zaftig opera star Jessye Norman, who filed a libel suit against *Classic CD Magazine* for portraying her as overweight (and uneducated); and Jane Bronstein, a large Connecticut woman, who is suing David Letterman for dubbing her "the peach lady" and repeatedly ridiculing her while showing film of her taken unaware at a tennis tournament with peach juice running down her chin.

Understand that, while many aspects of obesity are complicated, one thing is perfectly simple: civil and human rights should not depend on appearance.

Do the simple math that'll convince you that womanly sized women are not deviants; we are, in fact, the majority of the majority gender on this planet.

Now get angry. Angry enough to snap your puppet strings, and accept responsibility for your own recovery from the brainwashing. You can start by

- saying "No!" to the ventriloquists' voices inside and outside your head that say the only way to be attractive, or even socially acceptable, is literally to belittle yourself. Tip: Doing this is easier than it sounds, once you translate the code and understand that what these voices are *really* saying is "Give me your money";
- realizing that our society's obsession with extremely thin women, and our knee-jerk fear of fat, are as artificial as they are nonsensical, and did not "just happen";
- figuring out for yourself what your natural body weight seems to be, and what the most reasonable methods are for maintaining it— starting with the most realistic and reliable of all slogans in this context: If you can burn it, you can eat it;
- educating as many doctors as possible about the reality that "fat" and "fit" are not always mutually exclusive terms;
- refusing to accept appearance-based substandard treatment from anyone whose services you engage, be they physicians, hairstylists, clothing store clerks, or whatever;
- taking a similarly self-respecting stance with anyone who employs you;
- telling anyone who'll listen—and especially the audiences for phone-in talk shows—how the antifat profiteers manipulate us to meekly accept the premise that it's normal for women to literally go hungry;
- lobbying legislators and public-health officials for the introduction of appropriate regulatory measures (possibly including a Surgeon

General's report) that will—to borrow Susan Powter's vivid phrase—
"stop the insanity";

• contacting magazine editors to demand a halt to the onslaught of
"before-and-after" makeover articles that perpetuate the belief that
women must always be "fixed," and to point out how it would be in
their best economic interest to intersperse authentic images of
women among the nonstop depictions of what, for 95 percent of us,
are anatomical impossibilities;

• writing letters to editors of newspapers, and telephoning producers
of television and radio shows, asking them to explain how items such
as speculations about Princess Diana supposedly wearing long coats
to conceal flabby thighs can possibly be treated as genuine news;

• conversely, bombarding the media with positive reinforcement
when they do get it right in reports such as a recent attention grab-
ber in the *Wall Street Journal* to the effect that women are indeed
"dying to be thin" by smoking;

• stopping the entrenched habit of teaching young children that fat
is a taboo by shushing their innocent observations about large people;

• developing a repertoire of snappy retorts for whenever someone
criticizes your weight, or that of another woman. ("Why do you
care? Are you planning to bounce us on your knee? Take us up in
a hot-air balloon? FedEx us to Finland?");

• refusing to participate in the never-ending attitudinal beauty
pageant that pits woman against woman in a classic divide-and-
conquer strategy, while simultaneously stalling our progression
toward true social and economic equality;

• understanding that, for the sake of profit, our energy has been
diverted, our dreams have been dislodged, and our quests for fulfilling lives have been diminished to a single, senseless pursuit;

• reviving, in person and on the Internet, the kind of consciousness-
raising sessions feminists once used to work through their own psychological conflicts and to plot unified action to redress wrongs;

• "voting" with your dollars for products that have positive effects
on our physical and psychological health, and against those that
have negative effects. Remember that American women today have
tremendous purchasing power, especially because 75 percent of us
now work for salaries;

- comprehending that, to quote Naomi Wolf's admonition in *The Beauty Myth*, "We do not need to change our bodies, we need to change the rules."
- above all, working to transform a world where the saddest quote in this book, "If shame could cure obesity, there wouldn't be a fat person in the world," becomes obsolete, and the only remaining shameful attitude is intolerance.

If you need *more* provocation to become sufficiently outraged to do these things, consider the sheer enormity of the situation. During the shockingly brief span of three decades, the antifat juggernaut—which is the only major segment of public health that is completely unregulated—has transformed its own self-serving propaganda into a virtual religion that's sweeping the world. This gargantuan manipulation of public opinion and behavior is, I would argue, on a par with the advent and spread of Communism, and was accomplished by some of the same techniques, including mind control, peer pressure, and disinformation.

The smug moguls spearheading the billion-dollar brainwash are counting on women to continue behaving as vain, gullible, fearful fools. This strategy has always paid off in the past, and the high rollers are now gambling more than $100 million a year, in advertising costs alone, that it will also do so in the future. In fact, the monolithic H. J. Heinz Company, which owns Weight Watchers, has already prepared for a turn-of-the-century splurge by reserving ad space on the gatefold covers of several major magazines scheduled for January 2000.

That fat fighting will be an even bigger bonanza in the next millennium is such a strong corporate conviction that major conglomerates are globalizing at a furious pace. Nutri/System catapulted from the ashes of its 1993 bankruptcy by joining with some twenty-six other enterprises—including the mighty Johnson & Johnson health-care firm and a subsidiary of Japan's giant Fuji Bank—to develop an ambitious range of "wellness-oriented" products and services.

Weight Watchers is multiplying its international market lead in many countries, including France, where—against all odds—it is persuading formerly sensible *femmes* to swap their succulent cuisine for freeze-dried banalities. Elsewhere, WW is teaming up with a raft of insurers to inundate their millions of members with rebate offers on life insurance premiums. And its parent, Heinz, has bought up so many competitors that it recently leapt to command the number three spot in the $3.3 billion frozen-entrée industry.

Now enthusiastic imitators are finding inspiration in Heinz's double-dealing formula for capturing consumers coming *and* going, which was epitomized by another recent megadeal—with Eskimo Pie ice cream. Among these monkey-see-monkey-do companies is mammoth International Pizza, which encompasses Domino's franchises as far away as Poland. Its new venture: a coast-to-coast chain of weight loss centers.

Making all of this even more threatening is the recent escalation of media mergers. There was precious little safety in numbers in the past. But as more and more magazines, newspapers, broadcasters, and film-makers are swallowed up by fewer and fewer entities, the multiple voices we used to hear are being sucked into a mere handful of mono-lithic megaphones.

Corporate concentration is also all the rage in the fashion industry where, for example, a single company (LVMH Louis Vuitton Moët Hennessey) now owns Christian Dior, Givenchy, and Galliano, and is rumored to be acquiring Vivienne Westwood. And the cheek-by-jowl associations that now litter the food and tobacco worlds are exempli-fied by the ownership of General Foods (number one in the United States) by Philip Morris, plus R. J. Reynolds' acquisition of Kentucky Fried Chicken, Nabisco, Del Monte, and Chun King.

The incestuous result of all this is bound to be, not just the per-petuation of diet-till-you-drop propaganda adjacent to eat-eat-eat advertising, but also increased amplification of all the Big Lies that vic-timize women, and exclusion of the contrarian views and information that could produce a much healthier cultural climate.

Case in point: The British branch manager of the Omega watch company recently canceled an ad campaign in *Vogue* and declared a future boycott of the magazine. His motivation for doing so, said Giles Rees, was the "extremely distasteful and irresponsible" use of ultra-thin models. He had been particularly shocked by news that two of London's major modeling agencies had tried to recruit an anorexic fifteen-year-old patient at an eating-disorders clinic. Yet, even though his boycott was widely applauded, international behind-the-scenes negotiations to restore *Vogue*'s $50,000-plus ad campaign resulted in

Rees being overruled by higher-ups at Omega's multi-faceted Swiss headquarters.

Obviously, the pigheaded antifat profiteers are confident that women will *never* awaken from the hypnosis they induced so that they could pick $50 billion a year (and counting) out of our pockets. If their estimation of our idiocy is accurate, then our dream of achieving "ideal" bodies will continue to be the nightmare it became when the definition of attractiveness was set so thin it became a virtual impossibility.

Unless we wake up from this billion-dollar brainwash and begin thinking for ourselves, we will go on spending ourselves blind on false promises—and waging unwinnable wars within our own souls that undermine us psychologically, endanger us physically, and, ultimately, impoverish our entire society.

Acknowledgments

My abiding gratitude to my mother, Betty Postill, and my late grandmother, Margaret Anhorn, for functioning as dedicated "language cops" throughout my childhood;

to my sisters, Bonnie Cox, Louise Poirier, and Lynn Postill; my friends, Gay Claitman and Kent Bowman; my uncle, Ray Anhorn; and my parents, Betty and Bill Postill, for vital practical support;

to my friend, Beth Kaplan, and my editors at Birch Lane Press and Key Porter Books, for crucial creative support;

to Louisville attorney Brooks D. Kubik, for help with my chapter on employment discrimination;

to library personnel in Louisville and Toronto, for shepherding me through cyber labyrinths, as well as dusty historical avenues;

to many gallant women, for confiding painful memories, in person and via e- and snail-mail; and to numerous authorities, for providing insiders-only information;

to my agent, Helen Heller, for tracking me down and handing me an opportunity that rescued me from delusion and despair;

and to Betty Friedan, Gloria Steinem, Susan Faludi, Naomi Wolf, Susie Orbach, and many other feminist writers for guiding and inspiring me—long before, and while, I wrote *No Fat Chicks*.

Select Bibliography

Aburdene, Patricia and Naisbitt, John, *Megatrends for Women*, New York: Villard Books, 1992

Atwood, Margaret, *Lady Oracle*, New York: Simon & Schuster, 1976

Basinger, Jeanine, *A Woman's View: How Hollywood Spoke to Women 1930–1960*, New York: Alfred A. Knopf, 1993

Bennett, William, M.D. and Gurin, Joel, *The Dieter's Dilemma: Eating Less and Weighing More*, New York: Basic Books, Inc., 1982

Black, J. Anderson and Garland, Madge, *A History of Fashion*, New York: William Morrow & Co., 1980

Bordo, Susan, *Unbearable Weight: Feminism, Western Culture and the Body*, Berkeley: University of California Press, 1993

Brownmiller, Susan, *Femininity*, New York: Simon & Schuster, 1984

Brumberg, Joan Jacobs, *Fasting Girls: The Emergence of Anorexia Nervosa as a Modern Disease*, Cambridge: Harvard University Press, 1988

Chernin, Kim, *The Hungry Self: Women, Eating and Identity*, New York: Times Books, 1985

————. *The Obsession: Reflections on the Tyranny of Slenderness*, New York: Harper & Row, 1981

Clarke, Eric, *The Want Makers*, New York: Viking, 1988

Crossen, Cynthia, *Tainted Truth: The Manipulation of Fact in America*, New York: Simon & Schuster, 1984

Croteau, David and Hoynes, William, *By Invitation Only: How the Media Limit Political Debate*, Monroe, Maine: Common Courage, 1994

Douglas, Susan J., *Where the Girls Are: Growing Up Female with the Mass Media*, New York: Times Books, 1994

Dworkin, Andrea, *Pornography: Men Possessing Women*, New York: Putnam, 1981

Ellison, Ralph, *Invisible Man*, New York: Random House, 1947

Epstein, Diane and Thompson, Kathleen, *Feeding on Dreams: Why America's Diet Industry Doesn't Work & What Will Work for You*, New York: Macmillan Publishing Co., 1994

Ewen, Stuart, *All Consuming Images: The Politics of Style in Contemporary Culture*, New York: Basic Books, 1988

————. *PR! A Social History of Spin*, New York: Basic Books, 1996

Fallon, Patricia, Katzman, Melanie A. and Wooley, Susan, *Feminist Perspectives on Eating Disorders*, New York: Guilford Press, 1994

Faludi, Susan, *Backlash: The Undeclared War Against American Women*, New York: Crown Publishers, 1991

Ferree, Myra Marx and Hess, Beth B., *Controversy and Coalition: The New Feminist Movement Across Three Decades of Change*, Oxford, U.K.: Maxwell Macmillan International, 1994

Foster, Patricia (Ed.), *Minding the Body—Women Writers on Body and Soul*, New York: Doubleday, 1994

Fraser, Laura, *Losing It: America's Obsession With Weight and the Industry That Feeds on It*, New York: Dutton, 1997

Friedan, Betty, *The Feminine Mystique*, New York: W.W. Norton, 1963; New York: Dell Publishing, 1975

Green, Rosemary, *Diary of a Fat Housewife*, New York: Warner Books, 1995

Gross, Michael, *Model: The Ugly Business of Beautiful Women*, New York: William Morrow & Co., 1995

Guisewite, Mickey and Cathy, *Dancing Through Life in a Pair of Broken High Heels*, New York: Bantam Books, 1993

Hirschmann, Jane R. and Munter, Carol H., *When Women Stop Hating Their Bodies: Freeing Yourself from Food and Weight Obsession*, New York: Fawcett Columbine, 1995

Kaplan, Jane Rachel, *A Woman's Conflict: The Special Relationship Between Women and Food*, Englewood, New Jersey: Prentice-Hall, 1980

Laurence, Leslie and Weinhouse, Beth, *Outrageous Practices: The Alarming Truth About How Medicine Mistreats Women*, New York: Fawcett Columbine, 1994

Millman, Marcia, *Such a Pretty Face: Being Fat in America*, New York: W.W. Norton & Company, 1980

Mirabella, Grace, *In And Out of Vogue*, New York: Doubleday, 1995

Murphy, Robert F., *The Body Silent*, New York: Holt, 1990

Peters, Lulu Hunt, *Diet and Health with a Key to the Calories*, Chicago: Chicago Publishing, 1918

Polivy, Janet and Herman, C. Peter, *Breaking the Diet Habit: The Natural Weight Alternative*, New York: Basic Books, 1983

Roosevelt, Eleanor, *This is My Story*, Garden City Publishing, 1937

Rosenblum, Mort, *Who Stole the News?*, New York: John Wiley & Sons, Inc., 1993

Roth, Geneen, *When Food Is Love: Exploring the Relationship Between Eating and Intimacy*, New York: Dutton, 1991

Rubin, Theodore Isaac, M.D., *Alive and Fat and Thinning in America*, Coward, McCann & Geoghegan, 1978

Savan, Leslie, *The Sponsored Life: Ads, TV, and American Culture*, Philadelphia: Temple University Press, 1994

Schroeder, Charles Roy, *Fat Is Not a Four-Letter Word*, Minnetonka, MN:
Chronimed Publishing, 1992

Schwartz, Hillel, *Never Satisfied: A Cultural History of Diets, Fantasies and
Fat*, New York: The Free Press, 1986

Sears, Barry, *The Zone: A Dietary Road Map*, New York: ReganBooks, 1995

Seid, Roberta Pollack, *Never Too Thin: Why Women Are at War With Their
Bodies*, Englewood, NJ: Prentice Hall Press, 1989

Shorris, Earl, *A Nation of Salesmen: The Tyranny of the Market and the Subversion of Culture*, New York: W.W. Norton & Company, 1994

Stacey, Michelle, *Consumed: Why Americans Love, Hate, and Fear Food*,
New York: Simon & Schuster, 1994

Steinem, Gloria, *Moving Beyond Words*, New York: Simon & Schuster, 1994

Taylor, Elizabeth, *Elizabeth Takes Off: On Weight Gain, Weight Loss, Self-
Image & Self-Esteem*, New York: Berkley Books, 1987

Warren, Roz (Ed.), *Revolutionary Laughter: The World of Women Comics*,
Freedom, CA: The Crossing Press, 1995

Whiteside, Thomas, *Twiggy & Justin*, New York: Farrar, Straus & Giroux,
1967

Winfrey, Oprah and Greene, Bob, *Making the Connection: Ten Steps to a Better Body and a Better Life*, New York: Hyperion, 1996

Wolf, Naomi, *The Beauty Myth*, New York: Random House, 1990

Zerbe, Kathryn J, M.D., *The Body Betrayed: Women, Eating Disorders and
Treatment*, Washington, D.C.: American Psychiatric Press, Inc., 1993

Source Notes

Chapter 1: Discovering a Billion-Dollar Brainwash

5 Oprah wailed to her diary: Marjorie Rosen and Luchina Fisher, "Oprah Overcomes," *People*, January 10, 1994, p. 45

5 "Ninety-five per cent of dieters" regain all the weight they lost: renowned University of Pennsylvania study by Dr. Thomas Wadden, plus many other sources

6 "No one can make you feel inferior": Eleanor Roosevelt, *This Is My Story* (Garden City Publishing, 1937)

7 One-third of all North American women now 20 percent overweight: National Center for Health Statistics, "Fatter and Fatter" (editorial), *New York Times*, May 21, 1994, p. A14; 89 percent believe they're too heavy: Deborah Pike, "Mental Makeover," *Vogue*, May 1995, p. 291

9 Assigned story on a woman's lifelong obsession: Terry Poulton, "A Death by Denial," *Toronto Life*, February 1982, p. 27

10 " 'begging in beauty's disguise' ": Leonard Cohen, "The Singer Must Die"

10 Poulton's columns appeared in *Starweek* from 1983 to 1987.

10 Annual revenues of weight-loss industry estimated at $50 billion: "1997 Body Image Survey," *Psychology Today*, January/February 1997, cover story

11 Definition of "brainwashing": *The Random House Dictionary*, 1980 ed., p. 108

11 Poulton's classified ad published in *USA Today*: March 4, 1994, p. 5D

12 Lillian Russell weighed 200 pounds: Amy Irving, Sylvia Wallace, and David Wallechinsky, *The Intimate Sex Lives of Famous People* (Delacorte Press, 1981), p. 36

13 "the average weight of models, actresses, and beauty pageant contestants": Roberta Pollack Seid, *Never Too Thin: Why Women Are at War With Their Bodies* (Prentice Hall, 1989), p. 261

13 "nearly 30,000 women stated": "Feeling Fat in a Thin Society," survey by Drs. Susan and Wayne Wooley, University of Cincinnati College of Medicine, *Glamour*, February 1984

13 "would deliberately choose to be blind, deaf, or have a limb amputated": Natalie Angier and Gina Kolata, "Fat in America" series, *New York Times*, November 22–24, 1992, p. 1

14 "50 times more women in America suffering from anorexia or bulimia than are living with AIDS": Literature of National Association of Anorexia Nervosa and Associated Disorders (U.S.), Centers for Disease Control (U.S.) Surveillance Report, as of December 31, 1995

20 Most Boomers are thickening as they age: Shelly Reese, "Boomers Have Affluence With an Attitude," *Cincinnati Enquirer*, May 22, 1994, p. A7

20 "The almightiest dollars of all": Tracy Young, "Beauty and the Beat," *Allure*, February 1995, p. 109, and numerous other sources; " 'Eat, Drink and Be Merry' May Be the Next Trend," *New York Times*, quoted in "Running on Empty?" *Hartford Courant*, January 25, 1994

Chapter 2: The Incredible Shrinking Woman

23–26 Twiggy's arrival in New York: Thomas Whiteside, *Twiggy and Justin* (Farrar, Straus & Giroux, 1967), p. 4

24 Twiggy's weight and height: *Newsweek*, April 10, 1967, p. 62

24 " 'just like your next door neighbor if . . . skinny twelve-year-old boy' ": *New York Times*, March 20, 1967

24 *Women's Wear Daily* denounced: *Newsweek*, April 10, 1967, p. 63

25 Vreeland gushed: Whiteside, *Twiggy and Justin*, pp. 105–6

25 30 million teenage girls in America: Ibid., p. 64

25 " 'Whether the Twiggy look will now sweep . . . emaciating American teen-agers as it goes' ": *Newsweek*, April 10, 1967, p. 62

25 " 'It was a nightmare, trying to keep up' ": Michael Gross, *Model: The Ugly Business of Beautiful Women* (William Morrow, 1995), p. 179

25 Wilhemina's hummingbird diet: Ibid.

26 Jane Fonda admitted to a twenty-year eating disorder: Seid, *Never Too Thin*, p. 247

26 Sally Field developed bulimia: Marjorie Rosen, *"Eating Disorders:* A Hollywood History," *People* February 17, 1992, p. 97

26 1968 Miss America pageant protest: Myra Marx Ferree and Beth B. Hess, *Controversy and Coalition: The New Feminist Movement Across Three Decades of Change* (revised) (Maxwell Macmillan International, 1994), p. 42

27 *Woman from Willendorf* (also called *Venus of Willendorf*): *Encyclopedia Americana*, vol. 22, p. 543

27 Venus de Milo's measurements: Terry Nicholetti Garrison, *Fed Up! A Woman's Guide to Freedom* (Carroll & Graf, 1993), p. 21

28 Technological breakthroughs: J. Anderson Black and Madge Garland, *A History of Fashion* (William Morrow, 1980), pp. 194–5

28 Dressmakers' patterns invented: Norman King, *The Almanac of Fascinating Beginnings* (Carol Publishing Group, 1994), pp. 194–5

28 Charles Frederick Worth created salons: Black and Garland, *A History of Fashion*, p. 194 "employing live mannequins": Ibid, p. 191

29 Ready-to-wear clothing began to be manufactured: Stuart Ewen, *All Consuming Images: The Politics of Style in Contemporary Culture* (Basic Books, 1988), p. 75

29 Secular bibles piloted by Sarah Josepha Hale: "Sex, Lies & Advertising," in Gloria Steinem, *Moving Beyond Words* (Simon and Schuster, 1994), p. 153

29 " 'the American craze' ": Seid, *Never Too Thin*, p. 61

29 " 'Our willowy girls are afraid of . . . strikes us as a monster' " Harriet Beecher Stowe, quoted by Charles Roy Schroeder, *Fat Is Not a Four-Letter Word* (Chronimed Publishing, 1992), p. 49

29–30 Louise drank vinegar: Ibid.

30 Raison d'être of women's magazines: Steinem, *Moving Beyond words*, p. 154

30 " 'Perfect feminine beauty no longer . . . thinness was a necessary condition' ": Anne Hollander, *Seeing Through Clothes* (Viking Press, 1975), p. 154

30 " 'for the first time . . . a magazine had encouraged them to want' ": Steinem, *Moving Beyond Words*, p. 154

31 Sarah Bernhardt caricatured: William Bennet, M.D. and Joel Gurin, *The Dieter's Dilemma: Eating Less and Weighing More* (Bogie Books, 1982), p. 199

31 " 'Does your form lack . . . air form corset waist inflated to any desired size' ": Schroeder, *Fat Is Not a Four-Letter Word*, p. 59

31 " 'The hoop-skirt . . . all emblazoned in sartorial terms' ": Ibid., p. 53

32 "Edward Bernays . . . hold up Lucky Strike cigarette . . . 'torches of freedom' ": Stuart Ewen, *PR! A Social History of Spin* (Basic Books, 1996), pp. 3–4

32 " 'the rapidity with which the new, linear form . . . [was] startling' ": Hollander, *Seeing Through Clothes*, p. 154

32 " 'Women measure themselves . . . gobbled them up' ": Jeanine Basinger, *A Woman's View: How Hollywood Spoke to Women 1930–1960* (Alfred A. Knopf, 1993), p. 212

32 " 'there is one crime . . . than to be guilty of growing fat' ": *Vogue*, July 1, 1918, p. 78

32 " 'viewed with distrust, suspicion, and even aversion' ": Lulu Hunt Peters, *Diet and Health With a Key to the Calories* (Chicago Publishing, 1918), p. i

33 " 'quasi-scientific diet programs . . . special baths, pastes, and thinning salts' ": Joan Jacobs Brumberg, *Fasting Girls: The Emergence of Anorexia Nervosa as a Modern Disease* (Harvard University Press, 1988), p. 232

33 Adult Weight Conference: Ibid., p. 248

33 " 'To keep a slender figure ... Reach for a Lucky instead of a sweet' ": Patricia Fallon, Melanie Katzman, and Susan Wooley, *Feminist Perspectives on Eating Disorders* (Guilford Press, 1994), p. 413

33 "Lucky Strikes' targeting of women ... from third position to top brand": Bob Herbert, "Selling Sex and Cigarettes," *New York Times*, reprinted in *Courier-Journal* (Louisville, Ky.), January 3, 1996, p. B9

33 A million scales sold ...: Fallon, Katzman, and Wolley, *Feministive Perspectives on Eating Disorders*, p. 339

33 " 'We grew up founding our dreams on ... advertising' ": Zelda Fitzgerald, quoted by Diane Epstein and Kathleen Thompson, *Feeding on Dreams: Why America's Diet Industry Doesn't Work and What Will Work for You* (Macmillan, 1994), p. 10

34 " 'It is very little to me ... in my absolute right' ": Lucy Stone quoted by Andrea Dworkin, *Pornography: Men Possessing Women* (New York, Putnam, 1981), p. 11

34 Uneeda Biscuit: Earl Shorris, *A Nation of Salesmen: The Tyranny of the Market and the Subversion of Culture* (W.W. Norton, 1994), p. 53

35 "the savviest profiteers went right on developing": Dr. Paul Ernsberger and Paul Haskew, "Rethinking Obesity: An Alternative View of its Health Implications," special monograph published in *The Journal of Obesity and Weight Regulation*, Summer 1987, p. 42

36 " 'mirrored the yearning ... that existed for women then' ": Betty Friedan, *The Feminine Mystique* (W.W. Norton, 1963; Dell Publishing, 12th reprinting, 1975), p. 34

37 "crammed full of food ... the life of the mind and spirit": Ibid., p. 31

38 "The Fattest Girl in the Class": *Seventeen*, January 1948, pp. 21–2

39 "marketing had become a science": Shorris, *A Nation of Salesmen*, p. 191

39 "Working hand in glove ... had invented the classic techniques that endure today": Ewen, *PR! A Social History of Spin*, p. 157

39 Chronology of TV shows: Alex McNeil, *Total Television: A Comprehensive Guide to Programming From 1948 to 1980* (Penguin Books, 1980)

39 Market research a $2.5 billion industry: Leslie Savan, *The Sponsored Life: Ads, TV, and American Culture* (Temple University Press, 1994), p. 2

39 " 'Before television ... one of the forces that determined the world' ": Shorris, *A Nation of Salesmen*, pp. 89–91

39 " 'Behavior essential for economic reasons ... transformed into a social virtue' ": John Kenneth Galbraith, quoted by Michael H. Minton with Jean Libman Block, *What Is a Wife Worth?* (McGraw-Hill, 1984), pp. 134–5

41 " '[B]y promising to melt and float ... determined to be thinner": "Trapping the Obese," *Newsweek*, August 19, 1957, p. 60

41 "They Take Your Money, You Keep Your Weight," *Reader's Digest*, December 1959, p. 28

41 So many weight loss products belonged in snake oil category: "Trapping the Obese," p. 60

41 "part of the first generation of females": Friedan, *The Feminine Mystique*, p. 47

42 " 'the feminine mystique began to spread ... stranglehold on the future' ": Ibid., p. 37

42 " 'You just can't write about ... like the price of coffee' ": Ibid., p. 31

43 "Reduce the Way the Models Do": *McCall's*, July 1960, pp. 80, 118

43 Sucaryl ad: Ibid., p. 146

43 Five publications had perished: Friedan, *The Feminine Mystique*, p. 58

43 *Ladies Home Journal* taught a lesson: Steinem, *Moving Beyond Words*, p. 154

43 "ads had surpassed circulation sales as the top income source for most newspapers": Ewen, *PR! A Social History of Spin*, p. 87

44 "Chevrolet ... once censored the phase 'ford the river' ... the word "gas" cut out of the soundtrack of *Judgment at Nuremberg*": Eric Clarke, *The Want Makers* (Viking Press, 1988), p. 324

44 "McCall's ... devoted six pages ... and the brutal dictatorship of 'Papa Doc' Duvalier": A. Kent MacDougall, "Ladies' Home Journal, McCall's Fight It Out With Sugar and Spice," *Wall Street Journal*, August 3, 1970, p. 1

44 McCall's ads and complementary copy: Ibid., p. 157

44 " 'pulse to the ... patterns tend to fade away": Savan, *The Sponsored Life*, p. 5

45 "Weight Watchers had enrolled nearly 500,000": "Changing Lost Pounds Into Dollars," *Business Week*, March 4, 1967, p. 110

45 Weight Watchers techniques: quoted in *Business Week*, March 4, 1967, p. 111

45 " 'Creampuffs, there's no escape . . . stay that way' ": "The Tuned-Up Body," *Mademoiselle*, May 1970, pp. 175–6

45 $500,000 spent on "SweetaStakes": *Ladies' Home Journal*, July 1968, p. 11

45 "Inside I was Crying Until I Lost 150 Pounds": Ibid., September 1968, p. 64

45 Fleischmann's margarine ad: Ibid., p. 46

45 "How I Lost 80 Pounds . . . by a Governor's Wife": Ibid., October 1969, cover

45 $200 million "waistline industry": *Business Week*, March 22, 1969, p. 140

46 High school girls considered themselves too fat: Seid, *Never Too Thin*, p. 150

46 One in twelve girls vomit: Frances M. Berg, "Afraid to Eat: Children and Teens in Weight Crisis," *Healthy Weight Journal*, 1997, p. x

46 "Aren't you jealous . . . tells me her secrets": Fallon, Katzman, and Wooley, *Perspectives on Eating Disorders*, p. 408

46 "chubby dolls were 'ugly' ": Yale University study quoted in NAAFA (National Association for the Advancement of Fat Acceptance) literature

46 Teen suicides quadrupled in past three decades: Mary Nemeth, "An Alarming Trend," *Maclean's*, October 31, 1994, p. 15

46 " 'I can't take it anymore' ": "Student Kills Himself in Class in Cherokee," *Atlanta Constitution*, March 26, 1994, p. C4

47 An estimated 70 percent of American families using low-cal foods: Lois Anzelowitz, "You Call This Progress?" *Working Woman*, October 1992, p. 95

47 "physicians were by now prescribing some 10 billion amphetamines": Seid, *Never Too Thin*, p. 138

47 "Weight Watchers had spread to forty-nine states": "Fortune From Fat," *Time*, February 21, 1972, p. 71

47 First generation of liquid-protein resulted in three deaths: Anzelowitz, "You Call This Progress?"

47 Jane Fonda creating a one-woman fitness empire: W. Wolf, "Principles and Profits," *New York*, December 14, 1981, p. 90

47 $285 million spent on exercise videos: *People*, January 10, 1994, p. 36

47 Diet-food business was fastest-growing segment: "The Food Giants See the 'Light,' " *Business Week*, June 1, 1981, p. 112

47–48 Nestlé, Stouffer, and H.J. Heinz "mounting intensive ad campaigns": Ibid., p. 113

48 Liposuction resulted in twenty deaths yet became the most popular cosmetic surgery in history: Susan Faludi, *Backlash: The Undeclared War Against American Women* (Crown, 1991), p. 221

48 Liposuction leapt from zero to 250,000 operations by 1989: James Patterson and Peter Kim, *The Day America Told the Truth* (Prentice Hall, 1991), p. 54

48 First news story about anorexia: "Dieting Till Death," *Science Digest*, May 1970, p. 27

48 "a holdup . . . disrespect they have for women": Sey Chessler quoted by Gloria Steinem, "Sex, Lies & Advertising," *Ms.*, July/August 1990, p. 27

49 Pressures routinely exerted by marketers: Ibid., pp. 18–28

49 "revealed in her autobiography . . . ordered her to virtually ignore the health risks of smoking": Grace Mirabella, *In and Out of Vogue* (Doubleday, 1995), pp. 208–11

49–50 " 'revolution in marketing . . . with spending money' ": Michael Hoyt, "When the Walls Come Tumbling Down," *Columbia Journalism Review*, March/April 1990, pp. 35–41

50 " 'with newspapers facing tough times . . . criticizing advertisers in print' ": G. Pascal Zachary, *Wall Street Journal*, quoted by Jon Swan, "The Crumbling Wall," *Columbia Journalism Review*, May/June 1992, p. 23

50 " 'solicited advertisers first . . . feature them in [a] program' ": Joanne Lipman, *Wall Street Journal*, quoted ibid.

50 "McDonald's . . . gave the producers of *Santa Claus—The Movie* $1 million": Clarke, *The Want Makers*, p. 366

50–51 "the marketing budget for *Space Jam* soared to $70 million": Naomi Klein, "What's Up, Doc? Just Ask the Marketers," *Toronto Star*, November 18, 1996, p. A17

51 " 'they can now hijack our culture . . . choice is practically taken out of the equation' ": Ibid.

51 " 'The media may not directly . . . on what the public thinks about' ": David Croteau and William Hoynes, *By Invitation Only: How the Media Limit Political Debate* (Common Courage, 1994), p. 51

51 " 'favor impact over information . . . spread into a worldwide pandemic' ": Mort Rosenblum, *Who Stole the News?* (John Wiley & Sons, 1993), pp. 3, 9

51 Epidemic of eating disorders affects more than 11 million women and girls: National Association of Anorexia Nervosa and Associated Disorders (U.S.) literature; eating disorders affect 50 times as many North American women as are living with AIDS: HIV/AIDS Surveillance Report through December 31, 1995

52 " 'vomiting bathrooms' ": Kathryn J. Zerbe, M.D., *The Body Betrayed: Women, Eating Disorders and Treatment* (American Psychiatric Press, 1993), p. x

52 " 'bulimia parties' are now a popular pastime on campus": "U.S. College Program Battles 'Fad Bulimia,' " *Philadelphia Inquirer*, reprinted in *Toronto Star*, February 20, 1996, p. B3

52 " 'People were dieting long before . . . as did the Egyptians' ": Tina Gaudoin, "Body of Evidence," *Harper's Bazaar*, July 1993, p. 74

52 " 'Major advertisers . . . essentially "sell" the audience to advertisers' ": Croteau and Hoynes, *By Invitation Only*, p. 24

52 " 'Hey Coke, want 17 1/2 million very interested women . . . lively articles about staying in shape' ": *Advertising Age*, quoted by Fallon, Katzman, and Wooley, *Feminist Perspectives on Eating Disorders*, pp. 399–401

53 "What makes the whole situation even more insidious . . . including 350,000 commercials": Clarke, *The Want Makers*, p. 331

53 " 'the more we are bombarded . . . the more we are affected' ": Ibid, p. 13

53 "just three years after Twiggy's Manhattan triumph": "Twiggy to Retire as Fashion Model," *New York Times*, March 11, 1970, p. A7

54 "Jacqueline Kennedy . . . went on a diet": Susan Brownmiller, *Femininity* (Simon & Schuster, 1984), p. 48

54 "*McCall's* calling 'lib ladies . . . poor, strident, ridiculous, hung-up creatures' ": MacDougall, "Ladies' Home Journal, McCall's Fight It Out With Sugar and Spice"

54 "Two hundred feminist crusaders had stormed . . . occupying its office for eleven hours": John Mack Carter, "Women's Liberation and You: The Special Feminist Section Everyone's Been Talking About," *Ladies Home Journal*, August, 1970, cover story

55 " 'the feminist entreaty . . . quest for true self-determination' ": Faludi, *Backlash*, p. 71

55 " 'Ironically, as the role of women was redefined . . . the pressure to be thin' ": Seid, *Never Too Thin* p. 261

57 Sharp downturn in women's apparel sales and magazine subscriptions: Faludi, *Backlash*, p. 93

57 " 'Corporations saw . . . gold in them thar thighs' ": Susan J. Douglas, *Where the Girls Are: Growing Up Female With the Mass Media* (Times Books, 1994), p. 260

58 Weight Watchers' "taste of freedom" bread commercial: Fallon, Katzman, and Wooley, *Feminist Perspectives on Eating Disorders*, p. 405

59 1,500 images flicker before our eyes every day: Savan, *The Sponsored Life*, p. 2

59 Coca-Cola bottle redesigned: Ewen, *All Consuming Images*, pp. 179–80

59 Columbia Lady slimmed down: "Weight Watcher," *New Yorker*, August 16, 1993, p. 25

59 Saks Fifth Avenue's Grace Kelly–sized mannequins replaced: "Rat Patrol," *Working Woman*, April 1995, p. 9

60 Weight of actresses, etc., plunged: Seid, *Never Too Thin*, p. 261

60 Average weight and height of American women: Faludi, *Backlash*, p. 171

60 Actresses on *Friends* wear size 4: Marcia Harris, "White Girls Have Lots to Learn About Body Image," *Grand Forks* (N.D.) *Herald* reprinted in *Toronto Star*, January 7, 1997, p. E5, plus various other reports

60 Kate Moss's weight and height: Gaudoin, "Little Miss Moss," *Harper's Bazaar*, December 1992, p. 34

60 Height of supermodels: Charlotte Raven, "Super Models Icons for Young Women," *Guardian*, December 15, 1994, p. F4

60 " 'We now have cultural norms . . . our biological heritage' ": C. Wayne Callaway, M.D., quoted by Lori Miller Kase, "Weight Game," *Harper's Bazaar*, April 1993, p. 291

60 " 'feminine esthetic at odds . . . in its natural state' ": Susan Brownmiller, *Femininity* (Simon & Schuster, 1984), p. 48

61 "women now aspire 'not to look like the great beauties . . . and computer technique' ": Vicki Goldberg, "Advertisements for the Insecure, Unreal Self," *New York Times*, April 11, 1993

Chapter 3: A Mountain of Mendacity

63 " 'The secret of all true persuasion . . . take care of itself' ": H. A. Overstreet, *Influencing Human Behavior* (W.W. Norton, New York, 1925), p. 65

63 " 'When you control a man's thinking . . . and stay in it' ": Carter G. Woodson, quoted in the *Courier-Journal* (Louisville, Ky.), June 24, 1995, p A9

63 "majority of 33,000 female respondents declared": "Feeling Fat in a Thin Society" survey by Drs. Susan and Wayne Wooley, University of Cincinnati College of Medicine, *Glamour*, February 1984

63–64 "would willingly die five years younger": "1997 Body Image Survey," *Psychology Today*, February 1997, cover story

64 Eleven percent of respondents would opt to abort: Geoffrey Cowley, "Made to Order Babies," *Newsweek*, Winter/Spring 1990, p. 981

64 A decade and a half after Twiggy's debut, weight-loss industry profits were $10 billion: G. Ferry, "Food and Behavior," *World Press Review*, December 1983, p. 30

64 Annual revenues of weight loss industry quintupled to $50 billion: "1997 Body Image Survey," *Psychology Today*

64 "according to *Money* . . . up to $84 per pound *temporarily* lost": Andrea Rock, "Shrink Your Weight While Keeping Your Wallet Plump," *Money*, February 1997, p. 162

64 Most North Americans have gained weight in the past three decades: Patricia Chisholm, "The War on Fat," *Maclean's*, January 16, 1995, p. 46

64 "incredible Squee-Zer-Ciser . . . like rubber bands": Dave Barry column, syndicated in the *Toronto Star*, March 24, 1996, p. D16

64–65 "gadgets and gizmos": Donald Dale Jackson, "The Art of Wishful Shrinking Has Made a Lot of People Rich," *Smithsonian*, January 1986, pp. 150–6

65 Four million people tried liquid protein: reported in *Newsweek*, according to Bennett and Gurin, *The Dieter's Dilemma*, p. 238

65 U.S. Centers for Disease Control investigated fifty-eight deaths: Ibid.

65 " 'the full pink tint of a Beaujolais . . . only you can fail' ": Robert Linn, M.D., *The Last Chance Diet*, L. Stuart, 1976

66 Dr. Herman Taller convicted of mail fraud: Bennett and Gurin, *The Dieter's Dilemma*, p. 234

66 Dr. Robert Atkins called to appear before a congressional committee: Ibid.

66 " 'The more time you spend . . . the idea' ": Judy Mazel, *The Beverly Hills Diet* (Macmillan, 1980)

66 " 'any so-called hunger "pangs" . . . rather than true hunger' ": Allan Cott, M.D., *Fasting as a Way of Life* (Bantam, 1977)

66–67 "a scathing article . . . 'nutritionally unsound and probably dangerous' ": *Consumer Reports*, June 1993, cover

67 High attrition rates (35 to 40 percent) at fitness centers: Judith Newman, "Why We Don't Exercise," *Allure*, August 1995, p. 124

67–68 Techniques of TOPS and other weight loss clubs in early years: "Changing Lost Pounds Into Dollars," *Business Week*, March 4, 1967, pp. 110–11; and Donald Dale Jackson, "The Art of Wishful Shrinking . . .," *Smithsonian*, January 1986, pp. 150–6

68 " 'So what did you give yourself—a pot of fat?' ": Jackson, "The Art of Wishful Shrinking"

68 The pig song: Hillel Schwartz, *Never Satisfied: A Cultural History of Diets, Fantasies and Fat* (Free Press, 1986), p. 207

68 'Tapeworms are being marketed on the Internet': Susan Brink, "Pills, Balloons and Now Tapeworms," *Wall Street Journal*, August 7, 1995, p. 48
68 "Smart refrigerators, programmed to withhold snacks, are in development": "Brave New Fridge Curbs Overeating," *Daily Camera*, reprinted in the *Toronto Star*, January 2, 1997, P . E3
68 Sauna Shorts and Svelte-Patches: ad in *Starweek, Toronto Star*, April 20, 1996, p. K17
68–69 " 'I Watched My Neighbor . . . Didn't Call the Police' ": ad in *Woman's Day*, April 23, 1996, p. 29
69 "Japanese-manufactured seaweed soap . . . to lather fat away": *Wall Street Journal*, November 2, 1995, p. B1
69 Thigh creams to make unsightly cellulite vanish: *Tufts University Diet and Nutrition Letter*, February 1994, p. 3, and numerous other sources
69 "readers can 'reset [their] genetic code[s]' and 'eating fat doesn't make you fat' ": Barry Sears, *The Zone: A Dietary Road Map* (ReganBooks, 1995), cover flap
70–73 " 'no work, no muss, no fuss . . . smile on your face' ": Diane Epstein and Kathleen Thompson, *Feeding on Dreams: Why America's Diet Industry Doesn't Work and What Would for You* (Macmillan, 1994), p. 9
70 $50 million spent on January marketing spree alone: Kathy Tyrer, "The Big Weight Watch Is On," *Marketing*, January 31, 1994, p. 6
70 Counselors fired if they quote prices on telephone: Epstein and Thompson, *Feeding on Dreams*, p. 10
70–73 Costs and practices at commercial diet centers: Ibid., pp. 14–21
72 TV reporter took hidden camera to Jenny Craig: Author interview with Karen McCairley
72 Weight Watchers sells more than 250 food products: *Frozen Food Digest*, October 1995, p. 20
72–73 Weight Watchers' fees and practices: Epstein and Thompson, *Feeding on Dreams*, pp. 13–19
73 Weights-and-measures inspectors raided English reducing centers: Jane Gordon, "You're Only as Fat as You Feel," *Times* (London), April 5, 1996, p. 17
74 $77.6 million spent to launch Ultra Slim-Fast: "Nestlé Targets Dieters with New Chocolate Fix," *Advertising Age*, August 24, 1992, p. 6
74 Weight Watchers spent $40 million on ads: Tyrer, "The Big Weight Watch Is On"
74 Jenny Craig spent $50 million on ads: Ibid.
74–77 Biological basis for "Cro-Magnon Catch-22": Bennett and Gurin, *The Dieter's Dilemma*, and numerous other sources
75 Fewer calories than if we hadn't dieted: study by Dr. Rudolph Liebel, Rockefeller University, reported in *New England Journal of Medicine*, March 9, 1995
75 Conscientious objectors' experiment: Bennett and Gurin, *The Dieter's Dilemma*, pp. 11–16
76–77 " 'At Treblinka, 900 calories . . . sustain human functioning' ": Wolf, *The Beauty Myth*, p. 95
77 Discovery of "ob" gene: Natalie Angier, "Researchers Link Obesity in Humans to Flaw in a Gene," *New York Times*, December 1, 1994, p. A1
77 Fitness can result from thirty minutes of exercise per day: Panel of physiologists from the Centers for Disease Control and the American College of Sports Medicine, Stephen Brewer and Janis Jibrin, "Pound Foolery," *Modern Maturity*, May 1995; and numerous other sources

Chapter 4: Crazy or What?

79 Eleven percent of respondents would opt to abort: Geoffrey Cowley, "Made to Order Babies," Newsweek, Winter/Spring 1990, p. 98
80 "You snipe so steady / You snub so snide": Joni Mitchell, "Borderline"
83 " 'The thought of anyone parading naked' ": Suanne Kelman, "Fat in a Thin Society," *Chatelaine*, September 1993, p. 57
83 " 'How dare they impose that body on the rest of us?' ": *Love's Executioner and Other Tales of Psychotherapy*, Dr. Irvin Yalom (Basic Books, 1989), pp. 87–88
84 "bombarded with nonstop images" Steven J. Douglas, *Where the Girls Are: Growing Up Female With the Mass Media* (Times Books, 1994) p. 11

84 " 'we turn our bodies into metaphors' ": Jane R. Hirschmann and Carol H. Munter, *When Women Stop Hating Their Bodies: Freeing Yourself from Food and Weight Obsession* (Fawcett Columbine, 1994), p. 91

84 Average weight women believe they are too fat . . .: Thomas Cash, *What Do You See When You Look in the Mirror?: Helping Yourself to a Positive Body Image* (Bantam Books, 1995), quoted by Deborah Pike, "Mental Makeover," *Vogue*, May 1995, p. 291

85 " 'in every culture . . . more incidences of eating disorders' ": Martin E.P. Seligman, quoted in *Ladies' Home Journal*, April 1994, p. 56

85–86 Women suffer major depression at twice the rate of men: Leslie Laurence and Beth Weinhouse, *Outrageous Practices: The Alarming Truth About How Medicine Mistreats Women* (Fawcett Columbine, 1994), pp. 264, 275–6

85 Women are prescribed 83 percent of antidepressants, etc.: Ibid.

86 Chronic emotional distress doubles health risks: Daniel Goleman, *Emotional Intelligence* (Bantam, 1995)

86 " 'want to go away and hide' ": Judith Jordan, Ph.D., quoted by Natalie Tannen, "Heavy Soul," *Weight Watchers Magazine*, November 1994, p. 38

87 " 'I am invisible' ": Ralph Ellison, *Invisible Man* (Random House, 1947), p. 3

88 "When I'm Thin Fantasy": Geneen Roth, *When Food Is Love: Exploring the Relationship Between Eating and Intimacy* (Dutton, 1991)

89 Or check with the only . . . prime minister Kim Campbell . . .: Sydney Sharpe, *The Gilded Ghetto: Women and Political Power in Canada* (Harper Collins, 1994), p. 16

89 " 'Ronstadt has put on . . . pop star of the seventies' ": Karen Schoemer, "Linda Ronstadt: The Reluctant Superstar," *Mirabella*, April 1994, p. 58

90 " 'For a good part of my life' ": Patricia Foster, ed., *Minding the Body—Women Writers on Body and Soul*, as reproduced in *Toronto Life Fashion*, Fall 1994, p. 99

90 They'd rather be blind, deaf, or have a leg amputated: University of Florida study cited by Gina Kolata, "Fat in America," *New York Times*, November 22, 1992, p. 1

91 "the obese 'must be put in their place' ": Susan Bordo, *Unbearable Weight: Feminism, Western Culture and the Body* (University of California Press, 1993)

92 " 'exhibiting . . . weaknesses or flaws' ": Jane Rachel Kaplan, *A Woman's Conflict: The Special Relationship Between Women and Food* (Prentice-Hall, 1980), p. 7

92 "It is too bad that these women are begging to be left in their chains": Elizabeth Cady Stanton, in *Words of Women*, Anne Stibbs, ed. (market House Books, 1992)

92–93 " 'I've been acting differently,' " Jane R. Hirschmann and Carol H. Munter, *When Women Stop Hating Their Bodies: Freeing Yourself From Food and Weight Obsession* (Fawcett Columbine, 1995), p. 91

94 " 'I wake every morning hating myself' ": Marjorie Rosen and Luchina Fisher, "Oprah Overcomes," *People*, January 10, 1994, p. 45

94 "so ashamed of being 'the fattest woman in the room' ": Bob Greene and Oprah Winfrey, *Making the Connection: Ten Steps to a Better Body and a Better Life* (Hyperion, New York, 1996), pp. 1–2

94 Oprah was reluctant to accept Emmy award: Ibid.

94 " 'If shame could cure obesity' ": Dr. Susan Wooley, quoted by Dr. Judith Rodin, *Body Traps: Breaking the Binds That Keep You From Feeling Good About Your Body* (William Morrow, 1992), p. 89

95 " 'what was really starving' ": Elizabeth Taylor, *Elizabeth Takes Off* . . ., (Putnam's, 1987)

95–96 " 'collective worship at the shrine of slimness' " . . .: Brumberg, *Fasting Girls* p. 257

96 " 'profound humiliation that the body exists' ": Kim Chernin, *The Obsession: Reflections on the Tyranny of Slenderness* (Harper & Row, 1981), p. 50

96 " 'vomiting our guts out' ": Chernin, *The Hungry Self: Women, Eating and Identity* (Times Books, 1985), p. 8

96 " 'Restrained eating' ": Janet Polivy and C. Peter Herman, "Diagnosis and Treatment of Normal Eating," *Journal of Consulting and Clinical Psychology*, 1987

96 "Even 'normal' women have completely lost their perspectives" . . .: Quoted by Michelle Stacey, *Consumed: Why Americans Love, Hate, and Fear Food* (Simon & Schuster, 1994), p. 179

97 " 'The only way to get rid of temptation' ": Oscar Wilde, in *Bartlett's Familiar Quotations*, John Bartlett, ed. (Little, Brown, 16th ed., 1992), p. 566:14
97 " 'a myth that we can force our bodies' ": Louise Dickson, "It's Your Body, So Don't Abuse It," *Ottawa Citizen*, July 17, 1994, p. D6
98 Survivors of sexual abuse: Zerbe, *The Body Betrayed*, p. 201
98 "An inability to handle anger appropriately": Jane E. Brody, "Personal Health" column, *New York Times*, November 24, 1993, p. B9
98 " 'afraid that if I didn't eat' ": Chernin, *The Hungry Self*
98 " 'the one thing that will take care of me' ": Millman, *Such a Pretty Face: Being Fat in America* (W. W. Norton & Company, 1980), p. 109
98 " 'attempt to ward off depression' ": Rubin, *Alive and Fat and Thinning*, pp. 105–6
99 " 'Eating functions as a form of self-medication' ": Zerbe, *The Body Betrayed*, pp. 18, 30
99 " 'eating is the primary way of . . . maintaining human relationships' ": Peter Farb and George Armelagos, *Consuming Passions: The Anthropology of Eating* (Houghton Mifflin, 1980)
100 One-third of all Americans now at least 20 percent overweight: National Institute of Health for American literature
100 Christina Applegate "doubled over and passing out": Marjorie Rosen, "Eating Disorders: A Hollywood History," *People*, February 17, 1992, p. 97
101 Fat teenage girls less likely to be selected for top colleges: Jean Mayer, *Overweight: Causes, Cost and Control* (Prentice-Hall, 1968), p. 91
101 "stupidity, ugliness, and even mutilation preferable": "Growing Up Fat," *20/20*, ABC TV, July 28, 1995

Chapter 5: Doctor Feel-Bads

102 Some doctors are scribbling prescriptions for new diet "wonder drugs": daily ads for Diet Pharm in *Toronto Star* during 1997
103 17,500 "bariatric" physicians and 3,300 hospitals specializing in weight loss: Laura Fraser, *Losing It: America's Obsession With Weight and the Industry That Feeds on It* (Dutton, 1997), p. 198
103 "authorities officially declared that obesity is not merely a moral failing": Hirschmann and Munter, *When Women Stop Hating Their Bodies*, p. 97
103 " 'fat people are waddling reminders . . . blame the victim' ": Hillel Schwartz, *Never Satisfied*, p. 207
103 "majority of Americans are now overweight": Daniel Q. Haney, "Fat Americans in Majority for First Time, Survey Finds," Associated Press report, October 16, 1996
103 "health-care costs are estimated at a whopping $100 billion": Jennifer Warren, "Living Large," *Los Angeles Times*, December 27, 1994, p. E1
104 " 'fat people are blamed . . . victims than its perpetrators' ": Millman, *Such a Pretty Face*
104 "Shape Up America is largely funded by Weight Watchers": William J. Fabrey, "Big News" column, *Radiance*, Summer 1995, p. 46
104 $250,000 Heinz Award given to C. Everett Koop: *Courier-Journal* (Louisville, Ky.), December 1, 1995, p. 2
104 *Rump Parliament* published a cartoon of Koop as a hand puppet of the weight loss industry: Fabrey, "Big News"
104–105 Weight Watchers' membership is dropping: Janice Turner, "Are We Losing the War Against Losing Weight?" *Toronto Star*, June 19, 1995, p. A1; and Ellen Neuborne, "Slimmer Revenue Has Weight-Loss Industry Going on a Crash Diet," Gannett News Service, July 31, 1994
105 " 'Fat' and 'fit' are *not* mutually exclusive terms": Susan Carlton, "The Weight Debate," *Mirabella*, April 1994, p. 96, and many other sources
105–106 "One of my fellow panelists . . . locked up in prison camps": *Jane Hawtin Live*, WTN, October 11, 1996
106 Female patients talked down to, etc: Laurence and Weinhouse, *Outrageous Practices* p. 3
106 Doctors refuse to treat until weight is lost: Angier and Kolata, "Fat in America"
107 Raped woman traumatized, etc: Paul Ernsberger, "The Discriminating Doctor," *Radiance*, Fall 1988, p. 53

107 "Lose 50 Pounds and Call Me in the Morning" syndrome: Ibid.
107 "one third of family practice doctors admit to feelings of discomfort": Ibid.
107 Doctors' negative attitudes toward fat patients: D. Klein, J. Najman, A.F. Kohrman, and
    C. Munro, *Journal of Family Practitioners* (1982) 14:881–8.
107 " 'Unlike most "sick" people . . . why should I?' ": William Bennett, M.D., quoted in NAAFA
    literature
108 "restricting dietary carbohydrates so severely": Dr. Bryant Stamford, "The Body Shop,"
    Courier-Journal (Louisville, Ky.), March 15, 1994, p. C3
108 Elevated blood pressure, high cholesterol, etc., not caused by obesity: Janet Polivery and
    C. Peter Herman, *Breaking the Diet Habit: The Natural Weight Alternative* (Basic Books, 1983)
108–109 Relatively benign effect of excess weight on "pear-shaped" women: Jean-Pierre
    Despres, M.D., *Homemaker's*, March 1995, p. 131
109 Fat women eat less than thin women: *American Journal of Clinical Nutrition*, 1988, quoted
    by Ellen Hodgson Brown, *With the Grain* (Carroll & Graf, 1990), p. 22
109 Study of identical twins at Quebec's Laval University: Mary Louise Bringle, *The God of
    Thinness* (Abingdon Press, 1992), p. 122
109 Some degree of fatness is beneficial: Ernsberger, *Rethinking Obesity*
110 Complications and failure rates of weight loss surgery: Ibid.
111 Intestinal bypasses leapt from 30,000 to 50,000 in two years: Wolf, *The Beauty Myth*, p. 261
111 "Fibo pouch procedure": *Prime Time Live*, ABC, January 22, 1997
111 Even women whose weight was as low as 154 pounds: Fraser, *Losing It*, p. 198
111 Average cost of weight loss surgery: Ibid.
111 Liposuction's popularity drooped after complications and deaths: Pike, "Mental Makeover"
112 "27% Off Large Volume Liposuction" . . .: *Courier-Journal* (Louisville, Ky.), May 28, 1995,
    p. A13
112 "photographically bloated 'before' picture of Michelangelo's David": *Jewish Hospital Health-
    Care Services Newsletter*, Summer 1995, p. 16
112 Protein-sparing fasts cost $54.75 per pound: Rita Rubin, "The Cost of Weight Loss," *Amer-
    ican Health*, June 1994, p. 91
112 Amphetamines prescribed by the billions: Seid, *Never Too Thin*, p. 138
113 Fenfluramine may have caused brain damage in monkeys: Jane E. Brody, "Diet Drug May
    Harm the Brain," *New York Times*, May 11, 1994, p. C11
113 Dexflenfluramine caused deaths and incurable lung disease in France: *Prime Time Live*,
    ABC TV, May 8, 1996
113 Alarming *Time* cover story on Redux: Michael D. Lemonick, "The New Miracle Drug?"
    Time, September 23, 1996, cover
113 Risk of PPH soars to 3,000 per cent when taken for longer than three months: *New Eng-
    land Journal of Medicine* report reprinted in *Toronto Star*, August 29, 1996, p. A9
113 "average monthly cost of Redux is about $114": Associated Press report printed in *Courier-
    Journal* (Louisville, Ky.), April 22, 1996, p. 2
113 "Projections are that Redux will capture a $1 billion market share within five years": Lemon-
    ick, "The New Miracle Drug?"
114 American physicians have conflicts of interest: Sally E. Smith, "The Great Diet Deception,"
    USA Today, January 1995, pp. 76–78
114 North American Association for the Study of Obesity conference sponsored by . . .: Ibid.
115 Nutritional studies financed by Wonder Bread and M&M/Mars: Cynthia Crossen, *Tainted
    Truth: The Manipulation of Fact in America* (Simon and Schuster, 1994), p. 42
115 Researchers pre-sold thigh cream formula to Herbalife International: Paul Begoun and
    Kathy Jones, Knight-Ridder, printed in *Calgary Herald*, July 2, 1994, p. B6
115 FDA put Wyeth-Ayerst in charge of further clinical trials of Redux: Lemonick, "The New
    Miracle Drug?"
116 " 'a fundamental change in public thinking . . . a problem of willful misconduct' ": Institute
    of Medicine report quoted by Marlene Cimons, "Public Is Urged to Treat Obesity as Chronic
    Disease," *Los Angeles Times*, December 6, 1994, p. A14
116 " 'there is no commitment to obesity as a public health problem . . . on gluttony and
    sloth' ": William Dietz, M.D., "America the Bountiful," *New York Times*, July 19, 1994, p. A18

116 "There is an increasing number of . . . confines of established medicine.": Rubin, *Alive and Fat and Thinning in America*, pp. 27–29

Chapter 6: Hungry for Work

118 Sixty percent of overweight women denied employment: Angier and Kolata, "Fat in America" series, *New York Times*, November 22–24, 1992, p. 1

118 One-third of overweight women are routinely passed over for promotions and raises: Ibid.

118 Seventy-eight percent say rampant cruelty and injustice undermined confidence: Ibid.

118 Obesity results in $6,700 less per year: Doug Levy, "Obesity Affects Economic Health," *USA Today*, September 30, 1993, p. D1

118–119 NAAFA survey regarding employment discrimination: Angier and Kolata, "Fat in America"

118 "Overweight workers are penalized one thousand dollars . . . for every 'extra' pound' ": Ibid.

118 Thinnest fashion models are paid the most money: *Forbes*, March 27, 1995

119 " 'it's over for the 'fat lady' long before she sings' ": Nanci Hellmich, "Size, Gender, Income Linked," *USA Today*, July 13, 1994, p. 1

119 " 'We're running out of people that we're allowed to hate' ": Angier and Kolota, "Fat in America"

119 " 'The disabled serve as constant, visible reminders . . . a fearsome possibility' ": Robert F. Murphy, *The Body Silent* (Holt, 1990)

119 Attitudinal survey of 1,139 CEOs; and " 'I don't like fat people . . . opened his mouth' ": Judy Neuman, "Weighty Consequences of a Thin Argument," *San Jose Mercury News*, June 3, 1989, p. 1E

120 " 'Grossly overweight females are penalized more severely . . . same problem' ": Laurie Baum, "Extra Pounds Can Weigh Down Your Career," *Business Week* August 3, 1987, p. 96

120 " 'The American white relegates the black . . . nothing but shining shoes' ": George Bernard Shaw, quoted by Sharlene A. McAvoy, "Fat Chance: Employment Discrimination Against the Overweight," *Labor Law Journal*, January 1992, pp. 3–14

120 " 'The profundity of the narrowmindedness is incredible' ": Martin Everett, "Fat Chance," *Sales and Marketing Management*, March 1990, pp. 66–70

120 " 'I've had employers say to me . . . "has a flat stomach?" ' ": Elizabeth Kuster, " 'Lookism': The Workplace's Dirty Little Secret," *Glamour*, September 1993, p. 133

120–121 " 'Over the phone, they liked . . . never even considered.": Diane Wildowsky, quoted by Everett, "Fat Chance"

121 " 'Anyone who's supposed to . . . a big-time problem' ": Ibid.

121 " 'Managers assume that . . . lose them faster' ": Ibid.

121 " 'lazy, unkempt, jolly . . . and insecure' ": Ibid.

121 " 'most sales executives won't . . . field sales talent' ": Ibid.

121–122 " 'All fat people are "outed" . . . stay in my body'.": Jennifer A. Coleman, "Discrimination at Large ("My Turn" column), *Newsweek*, August 2, 1993, p. 9; and author interview

122 Business students hate being served by overweight people: Everett, "Fat Chance"

122 " 'If a business claimed that "fix" herself' ": Lindsy Van Gelder, "When Our Looks Aren't Good Enough," *Allure*, September 1992, p. 78

122 " 'Employers did not simply develop . . . calls itself a meriotcracy' ": Wolf, *The Beauty Myth*, p. 28

123–125 Blimpos Anonymous meeting: author interviews in Cincinnati, Ohio

124 " 'always to be doing work . . . my self, my soul' ": Virginia Woolf, *A Room of One's Own* (Hogarth Press, 1949)

126 *Krein v. Marian Manor Nursing Home* case: Sharlene A. McEvoy, "Fat Chance: Employment Discrimination Against the Overweight," *Labor Law Journal*, January 1992, pp. 3–14

126 Bonnie Cook case: Tamar Lewin, "Workplace Bias Tied to Obesity Is Ruled Illegal," *New York Times*, November 24, 1993, p. 1; Stephanie B. Goldberg, "Obesity," *American Bar Association Journal*, February 1994, p. 95; and numerous other reports

127–128 Toni Cassista case: Maura Dolan, "Job Bias Ruling Gives the Obese Limited Rights," *Los Angeles Times*, September 3, 1993, p. A1; " 'I started small . . . incorporated into the hiring process' ": *NAAFA Newsletter*, March/April 1993, p. 1

127 " 'a clear slap at the high court' ": David G. Savage, "Court Makes Job-Bias Suits More Difficult," *Los Angeles Times*, reprinted in *Courier-Journal* (Louisville, Ky.), June 26, 1993, p. 1

128 Santa Cruz public forum on appearance discrimination: *NAAFA Newsletter*, March/April 1993, p. 1

128 " 'I want an ordinance prohibiting . . . during daylight hours' ": Rush Limbaugh quoted ibid.

128–129 *Donoghue v. County of Orange* case: McAvoy, "Fat Chance"

129 " 'to make the tough decisions . . . outcasts and unhappy people' ": Ibid.

129 Nyleen Mullally case: *NAAFA Newsletter*, March/April 1993, p. 1

129–130 Sharon Russell case: Andrea Sachs, "Excess Baggage Is Not a Firing Offense," *Time*, March 25, 1991, p. 50; and numerous other reports

130 Flight attendants' battle: Daniel Seligman, "Fat Chances," *Fortune*, May 20, 1991; and numerous other reports

131 Actress had to lose 35 pounds to play an "ugly bitch": Rob Salem, "The Truth About Janeane Garofalo," *Toronto Star*, April 26, 1996, p. D1

131–132 Miss Universe's weight battles: "Miss Universe Works Out in Attempt to Lose Weight," Associated Press, printed in *Toronto Star*, February 1, 1997, p. K10

132 Trump called her "an eating machine . . . crown comes with absolute obligations": Trump appearance on *Entertainment Tonight*, February 5, 1997

132 Catherine McDermott versus Xerox: Jane Cooper, "Overweight and Under-Employed?" *Weight Watchers Magazine*, September 1990, p. 68; and McAvoy, "Fat Chance"

132 " 'It is significant to note . . . as a burden' ": McAvoy, "Fat Chance"

133 " 'the first red flag . . . claim-free labor force' ": Ibid.

133 " 'all too often . . . bad for the corporate image' ": William J. Fabrey, "The Discriminating Doctor," *Radiance*, Fall 1988, p. 53

133 " 'The extent to which . . . must be due to discrimination' ": Dr. Albert Stunkard, "Excess Baggage Is Not a Firing Offense," *New York Times*, November 22–24, 1992, p. 1

133–134 John Rossi awarded $1 million in damages: "Fired Obese Man Wins $1 Million," *Courier-Journal* (Louisville, Ky.), September 8, 1995, p. A5

134–135 U-Haul International "wellness" policies: McEvoy, "Fat Chance"

134 " 'barbaric . . . unconscionable . . . [and] outrageous' ": ACLU, quoted Ibid.

134 " 'more than half . . . implement such program [as U-haul's]' ": Ibid.

134 "an American will turn fifty every 7.5 seconds": Reese, "Boomers Have Affluence With an Attitude"

135 Coors and Hershey's "wellness" policies: McEvoy, "Fat Chance"

135 Class-action suit against Stouffer Foods: Ibid.

136 " 'an employer shall not: fail or refuse . . . weight or marital status' ": Michigan's Elliott-Larsen Civil Rights Act, quoted by Daniel Seligman, "Weightism," *Fortune*, May 25, 1987, p. 115

136 " 'one law too many' ": Governor Mario Cuomo, quoted in *NAAFA Newsletter*, May 1993, p. 7

136 " 'For too many years . . . must be ended' ": Assemblyman Daniel Feldman, quoted Ibid.

136 " 'We are a society that prides itself . . . regardless of body size' ": Sally E. Smith, quoted Ibid.

137 " 'It is my conviction that obesity is . . . ADA all about' ": Author interview with Coleman

137 " 'Protecting the obese . . . legislative intent' ": McAvoy, "Fat Chance"

137 Poulton's first job was at Great-West Life Assurance, Edmonton, Alberta, 1962

Chapter 7: Life With Laugh Track

140 "I don't want her, you can have her": "The Too-Fat Polka," Words and music by Ross Maclean and Arthur Richardson, © 1947

141 " 'Please don't feed the host' ": Clip from *Late Show With David Letterman* shown on *Oprah*, February 7, 1994

141 " 'the psychic scars caused by believing that you are ugly' ": Joan Rivers, *Quotable Women* (Running Press, 1989), p. 111

141 " 'like she devoured her previous husbands' ": Rivers, quoted by Roz Warren, ed., *Revolutionary Laughter: The World of Women Comics* (The Cross Press, 1995), p. 194

141 Fat jokes about Elizabeth Taylor: Rosemary Green, *Diary of a Fat Housewife* (Warner Books, 1995)

142 " 'Save the Males—Shave the Whale' " . . .: New York Times News Service, August 13, 1995

142 " 'death-row inmate is too fat to be hanged' ": Associated Press report, printed in the *Montreal Gazette*, September 20, 1994, p. F15

142 Forced a fat student to wear a "Wide Load" sign: reported in *USA Today*, April 28, 1994

142–143 " 'So, are you gonna take an ambulance' ": Ted Heusel, quoted by Bill Laitner, "Heavy Mettle," *Detroit Free Press*, May 5, 1995, p. 3F

143 " 'never met a meal she didn't like,' " etc.: Milton Berle, *Private Joke File* (Crown Trade Paperbacks, 1989)

144 " 'Quarter Pounder in one hand' ": Rachel Urquhart, "No-Sweat Exercise," *Vogue*, September 1994

144 " 'Where's the blubba, bubba?' ": "Diet Winners and Sinners," *People*, January 10, 1994, cover

144 "the latest reincarnation of the bygone circus fat lady": antics of the Jim Rose Circus described by Ira Band, "Gen X Circus Comes to Town," *Toronto Star*, February 27, 1997, p. G10

144–145 " 'nothing we humans like better' ": Daniel Pinkwater, "Portly's Complaint," *Omni*, April 1995, p. 103

145 ' "fear that our body will betray us . . . some can't' ": Author interview with Mark Breslin

146 " 'entered our living rooms . . . about her jeans size' ": *Revolutionary Laughter*, pp. 196–201

147 "A sleazy strip joint in the Midwest" is Deja Vu, in Louisville, Ky.

148 Comedians' habit of tacking on "ya fat pig": Author interview with Breslin

149 "Does Winfrey feel she's been punished": Clips from *In Living Color*, *Saturday Night Live*, *Seinfeld*, and *Late Show With David Letterman* shown on *Oprah*, February 7, 1994

150 " 'hips and thighs return to American couture' ": Wendy Wasserstein, "Goodbye Waif, Hello Bulge," *Harper's Bazaar*, November 1993, p. 86

150–151 Nauseating lima bean shake: *The Tonight Show*, May 1, 1995

151 Los Angeles's mythical antifat laws: *Greg Kinnear Show*, August 8, 1995

151 " 'The reason men will never understand' ": Mickey and Cathy Guisewite, *Dancing Through Life in a Pair of Broken High Heels* (Bantam Books, 1993), pp. 21–22

151–152 Adbusters' "Calvin Swine" bulimia ad: Author interview with Kalle Lasn and Linda Gould

Chapter 8: Starved for Affection

154 Courtship of Lillian Russell by Diamond Jim Brady: Irving, Wallace, and Wallechinsky, *The Intimate Sex Lives of Famous People*; Fraser, *Losing It*, p. 21

154 " 'sonnets of motion' ": Bennett and Gurin, *The Dieter's Dilemma*, p. 200

156 "just a sham to get the man a 'green card' ": *L.A. Law*, April 16, 1992

157 Fat Chicks ranked below cocaine users, etc: Warren, "Living Large"

157 "large women are least 20 percent less likely to marry": Doug Levy, "Obesity Affects Economic Health," *USA Today*, September 30, 1993, p. D1, quoting a study reported in the *New England Journal of Medicine*

157 " 'forced into celibacy' ": Ann Landers, Creators Syndicate, March 21, 1995

157 "attempting to have his wife killed": *Virginian-Pilot*, February 7, 1990, p. A5

158 "They Hate Me Just Because I'm Fat": *Carnie*, Fox TV, September 6, 1995

158 " 'weight as the central issue of their lives' ": Seid, *Never Too Thin*, p. 29

158 " 'to tell a woman she is ugly' ": Wolf, *The Beauty Myth*, p. 361

158–159 " 'the next thing you know, you're a ghost' ": Whitney Otto, *Now You See Her* (Villard Books, 1994), p. 296

159–160 Doctor traded stomach stapling for sex: "Sex Abuse Costs Doctor His Licence," *Toronto Star*, April 26, 1996, p. A7

160 " 'I couldn't say no to my husband' ": Hirschmann and Munter, *When Women Stop Hating Their Bodies*, p. 284

160 " 'the size of three ordinary thighs' ": Margaret Atwood, *Lady Oracle* (Simon and Schuster, 1976), p. 121

160–161 ' "I just shut down' ": Leslie Lampert, "Can a Woman Be Fat and Happy? *Ladies' Home Journal*, March 1995, p. 123

161 " 'spent more time in bed pulling our stomach in' ": Laura Fraser, "A Critic Looks at Pornography From the Inside," *Extra!* July/August 1993, p. 19

161 How to pose in bed so you won't look fat: *Cosmopolitan* magazine article, quoted by Wolf, *The Beauty Myth*, p. 201

161 Fully 90 percent of women feel bad about their bodies: Eating Disorders Centre literature

161 " 'The tyranny of the ideal image . . . learn to hate ourselves' ": Fallon, Katzman, and Wooley, *Feminist Perspectives on Eating Disorders*, p. 396

163 " 'My Husband Fell in Love With a 'New' Woman, and It Was Me!": *Shape*, September 1996, p. 124

163 " 'The need to be extraordinarily beautiful' ": Millman, *Such a Pretty Face*, p. 220

163 " 'don't see things as they are' ": Anaïs Nin, quoted in *Quotable Women* (Running Press, 1989), p. 76

163 Women would give up their husbands, boyfriends, careers, and money: *Vogue*, 1989, quoted by Schroeder, *Fat Is Not a Four-Letter Word*, p. 201

164 " 'my hormones started bubbling' ": Ibid., p. iv

164 "who could possibly be interested in marrying her": Rebecca Salner, "A Search for Size Acceptance: Big People Whittle Away at Social Indignities," *San Jose Mercury News*, August 8, 1988, p. 1A

164 Denounces "worship of the too-thin, childlike female body": Ken Mayer, *Real Women Don't Diet: One Man's Praise of Large Women and His Outrage at the Society That Rejects Them* (Bartleby Press, 1993), p. 168; appearance on *Donahue*, February 24, 1995

164 " 'I think I'm a throwback": Mayer, as quoted by Carla Wheeler, "Don't Diet," Gannett New Service, February 1, 1994

165 " 'Fat women are often harder to approach' ": Dan Davis, *Radiance*, Summer/Fall 1986, p. 20

165 " 'we are missing the humanity in people' ": Kathy Bates, quoted by Jeff Hayward, *Chicago Tribune*, May 14, 1995

166 " 'an enormous, life-altering mistake' ": Roth, *When Food Is Love* p. 97

Chapter 9: Dumped by Design

167 "Any demographer could have told them": Faludi, *Backlash*, p. 171

167–168 "spurning . . . an estimated 40 million consumers, who had a combined buying power of $6 billion": Jolie Solomon, "Fashion Industry Courting Large Women," *Wall Street Journal*, September 27, 1985, p. 32

168 Princess Elizabeth and the Duchess of Windsor denounced the retrogression: Jeanne Perkins, "Dior," *Life*, March 1, 1948, p. 84

168 Rebellion against Christian Dior's "New Look": Ibid., and "Counter Revolution," *Time*, September 15, 1947, p. 87

168 "the lucrative New Look swept to supremacy": Ibid.

169 more American women were working outside the home than remaining in it": Mirabella, *In and Out of Vogue* (Doubleday, 1995), p. x

170 " 'Well, they eat a lot . . . So why not give them polyester?": Terry Poulton, "Plump Profits," *Canadian Business*, June 1978, p. 54

170 " 'added up to a big yech' ": Una Abramson, *Chatelaine*, September 1970, p. 84

171 " 'fashion came to be about nothing more than' ": Mirabella, *In and Out of Vogue*, p. 14

172 "80 percent of women had come to detest": Faludi, *Backlash*, p. 170

172 Women spent more on houses, cars, and restaurant meals: Ibid.

173 "might misportray the fashion world as 'a nightmarish cartoon' ": Martha Duffy, "Fashion's Fall," *Time*, April 25, 1994, p. 50

173 " 'We'd describe [Kate Moss] . . . to describe Twiggy back in 1967' ": John Leland, "Back to Twiggy," *Newsweek*, February 1, 1993, p. 64

173 "waifs looked like 'angelic little boys' ": Elizabeth Tilberis, quoted by Amy M. Spindler, "How Fashion Killed the Unloved Waif," *New York Times*, September 17, 1994, p. B13

173 "Foisted all this bunkum . . . and then wondered why subscriptions were sagging": Mirabella, *In and Out of Vogue*, p. 184

174 "Scuttling together 'like characters in an Agatha Christie novel' ": Spindler, "How Fashion Killed the Unloved Waif"

174 Wintour "discovered" what she termed the switch to "Strong and Sexy" (*Vogue*, May 1994), quoted Ibid.

174–175 " 'A lot more people will be thanking us' ": Elizabeth Tilberis, quoted Ibid.

175 " 'suggest[ing] prostitution [and] sadism' ": Barbara Lippert, *Adweek*, October 3, 1994, p. 54

175 " 'Notice my breasts before . . . go long on pork-belly futures' ": Margaret Carlson, *Time*, transmitted on America OnLine 94-04-01

175–176 While regular-size sector was sinking, plus-size market was enjoying double-digit growth: U.S. Commerce Department report, quoted by Patricia Aburdene and John Naisbitt, *Megatrends for Women* (Villard Books, 1992), p. 206

176 Shaw began raising consciousness by marching into buyers' offices: Mary Peacock, "The Fashion Industry Courts 'The Big Woman' " *Ms.*, June 1980, p. 83

176 "They'd read a decisive demographic study": Ibid.

176 " 'they noticed we had that green stuff in our fat little fists' ": Solomon, "Fashion Industry Courting Large Women"

177 Oscar de la Renta and several other biggies designed for the Barbie doll: S. Shapiro, "My Mentor, Barbie," *New York Times*, November 6, 1994, p. 8

178 "far from being aberrant or inconsequential": National Institute for Health-Related Statistics report, quoted by Stephania H. Davis, "We're All Getting Bigger and So Are Our Fashions," *Hartford Courant*, July 31, 1994

178 Those who served Fat Chicks shared in a market bonanza: Jane Milstead, "Grandes Dames," *Los Angeles Times*, July 10, 1994, p. 26

178 "Bacon's took the virtually unprecedented step": *Courier-Journal* (Louisville, Ky.), June 18, 1995, p. A3; and author interview with Bacon's spokesperson

178 " 'They finally found out that we're not just . . . doctors and lawyers and businesswomen' ": Lisa Respers, "Big Clothing Has Been a Bright Spot in the Struggling Industry," *Los Angeles Times*, October 25, 1994, p. D1

178 " 'I can go shopping now and find' ": Gaile Robinson, "Big Gets Beautiful—Finally," *Los Angeles Times*, August 14, 1992, p. E1

179–181 Jackqueline Hope's "Big, Bold & Beautiful" story: Author interview with Jackqueline Hope

181 "number of suppliers of plus-sizes has leapt from 200 to over 2,000 in the past seven years": "Reality Check," *Mode*, Spring, 1997, p. 48

181 " 'Dressing is . . . a process of self-creation' ": Seid, *Never Too Thin*, p. 44

182 "Serious research is finally being done into the dimensions": Angela Bonavoglia, "What's Ms. Doing at the Fall Fashion Shows?," *Ms.*, September/October 1995, p. 53

182 "coming up with same kind of standard sizing men enjoy": Judith Egerton, "Custom-made Clothing Growing on Consumers," *Courier-Journal* (Louisville, Ky.), February 7, 1995, p. C1

183 1647 shop named in honor of the 47 percent of British women who wear size 16: Karin Davies, " 'Fashionably Fat' Briton Stumps for the Plump," *Los Angeles Times*, June 19, 1994, p. A21

183 Computer magic to make models look larger: Cara Wall, "FashionFax," *Glamour*, September 1993, p. 216

184 " 'There is still enormous prejudice among retailers when it comes to plus sizes' ": Alan Millstein, quoted by Alex Witchel, "Size 14, 190 Pounds: A Model Figure," *New York Times*, March 12, 1997

184 Simply upsized garments and left skinny little numbers in place: Wall, "FashionFax"

184 Standard size-10 dress forms have been inflated: Ibid.

186 " 'elongated to death' ": Karl Lagerfeld, quoted in *Women's Wear Daily*, reprinted in *Toronto Star*, July 11, 1996, p. C2

186 Corsets receiving unanimous support again: "Waist Case," *Vogue*, September 1994, p. 244

186 " 'The days when women followed fashion blindly are over' ": Aburdene and Naisbitt, *Megatrends for Women*, p. 205

Chapter 10: Fed Up

188 "outposts in your head": Sally Kempton, "Cutting Loose," *Esquire*, July 1970

188 " 'A quietly mad population is a tractable one' " . . .: Wolf, *The Beauty Myth*, p. 187

189–190 "virtually endorsed bulimia as normal beauty imperative": Gaudoin, "Body of Evidence"

190 Graffiti campaign defaced Calvin Klein jeans ads: Stuart Elliott, "Group Seeks Boycott of Calvin Klein," *New York Times*, May 4, 1994, p. D20

191–192 NAAFA twenty-fifth anniversary march on Washington: Gannett wire service report, August 26, 1994
192 " 'government has become a veritable food fight' ": Carl Weiser, Gannett News Service report, August 26, 1994
192 "what he apparently thought was a humorous kicker": Scott Harris, "Fighting the Battle for Fat Liberation," *Los Angeles Times*, March 30, 1995, p. B3
193 Statements by David Boaz and Laird Wilcox: Carl Weiser, Gannett News Service report, August 26, 1994
193 " 'Got a weight problem . . . phone Uncle Sam' ": Margaret Carlson, "And Now, Obesity Rights," *Time*, January 7, 1994
194 "One of Smith's personal bests": Smith, "The Great Diet Deception"
197 NAAFA threatened to boycott Denny's restaurants: William Fabrey, "Big News," *Radiance*, Fall 1994, p. 60
197 "Boycott Anorexic Marketing (BAM) began targeting": Elliott, "Group Seeks Boycott of Calvin Klein"
197 National Organization for Women (Los Angeles chapter) endorsed BAM: Ibid.
197 "Wyden . . . declared that "[m]illions of Americans abused . . . for all the good they get' ": Fraser, *Losing It*, p. 220
197–198 Crackdowns resulted from Senator Ron Wyden's congressional hearings: "Reins Tightened on Diet Aids," *Environmental Nutrition*, March 1994, p. 1, and Smith, "The Great Diet Deception"
198 "Institute of Medicine issued a . . . statement urging the weight loss industry 'to disclose the true effectiveness of its programs' ": Associated Press wire report, December 6, 1994
199 "National Education Association is currently investigating size discrimination in public schools": Joanne Ikeda, R.D., "Confessions of a Radical Registered Dietitian," *Radiance*, Spring 1995, p. 46
200 " 'Watch out, thin people' ": Alice Ansfield, ". . .," *Radiance*, Fall, 1988, p. 2
201 Trivialized complaints about her column: Diane White, "Fat Chance of Recruiting Yours Truly," *Boston Globe*, August 18, 1990, p. C7
201 "Ugly Fattie Weighs in Against Bulge Battle": *Barrie* (Ontario) *Examiner*, November 13, 1996
202 " 'I feel ashamed of my culture' ": Leslie Lampert, "Fat Like Me," *Ladies' Home Journal*, May 1993, p. 154
202 " 'You can't tell a person's fitness level by his appearance' ": Florence Griffith Joyner, "Fitness with Foreman and Flo-Jo," *USA Weekend*, September 8–10, 1995, p. 14
202–203 "wangled her way into a profit-making seminar": Laura Fraser, "Dieting by Prescription," *Vogue*, May 1995, p. 182
203 " 'Refuse to be nameless, depersonalized, manipulated' ": Friedan, *The Feminine Mystique*, p. 298

Chapter 11: Dying to Be Thin

204–213 The Juliette Christie story: Poulton, "A Death by Denial"
214 "Hush money" from plaintiffs keeps mortality rates secret: Frances M. Berg, "Sudden Death Syndrome Continues to Chill Treatment Centers," *Healthy Weight Journal*, May/June 1994, p. 51
215 "Diet pills containing . . . 'fen-phen' combination were blamed . . . seventy-eight incurable cases of PPH": *Prime Time Live* ABC, May 8, 1996
216 "Thirty heart attack deaths were attributed to . . . the Cambridge Diet": Fraser, *Losing It*, pp. 91–92
216 "Two dozen deaths have resulted from herbal diet potions": Ibid., pp. 94–99
216 "Nine women died in France . . . at least twenty deaths": Faludi, *Backlash* p. 221
217 " 'One of the fundamental tenets of the weight loss industry . . . and be better off' ": Steven N. Blair, "Harvard Alums Risk Disease by 'Always' Dieting," *Healthy Weight Journal*, May/June 1994, p. 52
217 Most likely causes of death . . .: Ibid.; also "Low-Calorie Diets Carry Some Risks, Physicians Warn," Chicago Tribune, January 5, 1990, and author interviews with various authorities

217 At least fifty-eight deaths have been blamed on liquid-protein diets: U.S. Centers for Disease
Control and Prevention report, quoted by Bennett and Gurin, *The Dieter's Dilemma*, p. 238
218 Epidemic of eating disorders compared with AIDS/HIV: Literature of National Association
of Anorexia Nervosa and Associated Disorders, Centers for Disease Control and Prevention
Surveillance Report, as of December 31, 1995
218 Jane Fonda forced herself to throw up twenty times a day: Rosen, "Eating Disorders: A Hollywood History"
219 Anonymous conjecture about Mama Cass Elliot's death proven false by an autopsy: Fraser,
Losing It p. 240
219–221 Details of Mama Cass's crash diet and its consequences: Cass Elliot, "What a Way to
Diet," *Ladies' Home Journal*, March, 1969, p. 76
220 " 'proof that one didn't have to be beautiful' ": obituary, *New York Times*, July 30, 1974, p. 36
220–221 Details of Mama Cass's influence and comeback attempt at Caesar's Palace: William
Kloman, "Sink Along With Mama Cass," *Esquire*, June, 1969, p. 102

Chapter 12: Belly-Up?

224 Many women would willingly accept early death in return for being thin: "1997 Body Image
Survey," *Psychology Today*, cover story
226 " 'Twiggy couldn't have arrived at any other time' ": Diana Vreeland, quoted by Whiteside,
Twiggy and Justin, p. 117
228 Someone will turn fifty every 7.5 seconds: Reese, "Boomers Have Affluence With an Attitude"
229 Number of chronic American dieters dropped from 65 to 48 million: Calorie Control Coun-
cil, quoted by Lori Miller Kase, "Weight Game," *Harper's Bazaar*, April 1995, p. 291
229 Drop in thinking "overweight" automatically means "unattractive": Adler, "The Joys of Living Large"
229 Rather win a Pulitzer Prize than be Miss America: Anna Quindlen, "1990s Feminism: Babes
or Sisters," *New York Times*, January 20, 1994
229 Aren't automatically making dieting number one New Year's resolution: University of Pennsylvania study, reported in *Bottom Line* newsletter, February 15, 1994, p. 8
229 1,900 new low- and no-fat food products introduced in 1995: "What's New at Mealtime?"
USA Weekend, November 8–10, 1996, p. 9
229 "The most admirable effort": Kellogg's Special K ads appeared in several issues of, among
other periodicals, *Chatelaine* and *Homemakers*
230 " 'I've done everything I could do . . . without being arrested' ": Calvin Klein, quoted by John
Leo, "Selling the Woman-Child," *U.S. News and World Report*, June 13, 1994, p. 27
230 Calvin Klein withdrew a major ad campaign for the first time: Richard Martin, "The Ultimate Fashion Taboo," *Los Angeles Times*, September 3, 1995, p. M2
230 "Food is good" campaign in Milan: Robin Givhan, *Washington Post*, reprinted in *Toronto
Star*, October 10, 1996, p. J4
231 Steven Spielberg to produce *Body Language*: "Weight Watch," *Entertainment Weekly*, July
29, 1994, p. 13
231 " 'craftiest, funniest and sexiest art around' ": *Newsweek*, quoted in *Toronto Star*, December
22, 1996, p. E2
232–233 " 'I'm a big, healthy woman with sturdy feet' ": Brett Butler, quoted in *Entertainment
Weekly*, October 7, 1994
233 " 'I don't think that I'm less of a person . . . better when I'm thinner' ": Rosie O'Donnell
quoted in *Ms.*, January/February, 1997, p. 53
234 "featured Rosie O'Donnell on its cover . . . on top of her thighs": *Woman's World*, April 6,
1997, cover
235 Wrote to Dear Abby and littered her book with self-degrading remarks: Green, *Diary of a
Fat Housewife*, pp. 25, 322
235–236 " 'superior to fat people' ": Helen Gurley Brown, *The Late Show* (William Morrow,
1993), pp. 87, 155
236 " 'still socially and legally acceptable to call someone a "big fat dope" ' ": Author interview
with Dr. Moe Lerner

236 Pam Hollowich sued Southwest Airlines: Warren, "Living Large"

236 Tobacco marketers spend $6 billion a year on advertising: Kathleen Kenna, "U.S. Butting Out for Camel and Marlboro Man," *Toronto Star*, February 8, 1997, p. C1

236 Teenage girls are the fastest growing segment of 3,000 American teenagers who begin smoking every day: Lynda Dexheimer, "Puff Pieces: Magazines Increasingly Feature Smoking," Gannett News Service, May 7, 1995; Elizabeth Gleick, "Now Joined by Clinton, Local Crusaders Against Teen Smokers Are Gaining Ground": *Time*, transmitted on America OnLine August 13, 1995

237 "obesity has more than doubled in the six-to-seventeen age group": National Center for Health Statistics survey, quoted in the *Washington Post*, October 3, 1995

237 "The average child sees 10,000 food commercials a year": Kelly D. Brownell quoted by Jim DeBrosse, "The Out-of-Shape Union: America Growing Under Weight Crisis," Cox New Service, *Courier-Journal* (Louisville, Ky.), May 29, 1997, p. F5.

238 90 percent of all American girls ages 3–11 own one or more Barbie dolls: Anna Quindlen, "Barbie at 35," *New York Times*, September 18, 1994

239 Jessye Norman suing Classic CD Magazine for libel: *Toronto Star*, November 1, 1995, p. D2

239–240 "Peach Lady" suing David Letterman for ridiculing her: Associated Press report in *Toronto Star*, February 6, 1996, p. C4

241 Princess Diana supposed . . . treated as genuine news: Reuters wire service report published in the *Toronto Star*, April 10, 1995, p. A5

241 Women are "dying to be thin": *Wall Street Journal*, reprinted in the *Toronto Star*, as "Are Smokers Dying for Smaller Dress Size?" April 1, 1996, p. B3

242 Weight-loss industry is spending $100 million on advertising: Kate Fitzgerald, "Weight-Loss Biz May Get Crash Diet," *Advertising Age*, May 10, 1993, p. 3

242 H. J. Heinz has reserved ad space for January 2000: "Creative Media Plans Ahead," *Inside Media Online*, transmitted April 26, 1995

242 Nutri-System catapulted from bankruptcy and joined twenty-six other enterprises: Richard A. Melcher, "Care and Feeding at Nutri/System," *Business Week*, March 7, 1994; including a subsidiary of Fuji Bank: Bill Laitner, "Susan Powter Gets Into Diet Business She Bashed," *Detroit Free Press*, May 18, 1995; and Johnson & Johnson: "Venture by Nutri-Systems," *New York Times*, March 5, 1994, p. 27

242 Weight Watchers' foods gaining success in France: "*Weight Watchers veut peser plus lourd*," *Tribune DesfossessOS*, March 7, 1995, p. 12

242–243 Weight Watchers teaming up with life insuers: Keith L. Alexander, "A Health Kick at Weight Watchers," *Business Week*, January 16, 1995

243 "Heinz . . . recently leapt to command the number three spot": Ibid.

243 Weight Watchers' megadeal: Chip Jones, "Richmond-Based Eskimo Pie to make Treats for Weight Watchers," *Richmond Times-Dispatch*, January 24, 1995

243 International Pizza owns Domino's franchises as far away as Poland, and is venturing into operating weightloss centers: *ABI Business NewsBank*, December 1, 1994

243 Media mergers are threatening: "Media Merger Mania" (editorial), *New York Times*, September 2, 1995; and numerous other sources

243 "Corporate concentration is . . . acquiring Vivienne Westwood": Bernadette Mora, "Fashion Notebook," *Toronto Star*, September 26, 1996, p. J2

243 "And the cheek-by-jowl associations": Mirabella, *In and Out of Vogue*, p. 207

243–244 Omega watch company's ad campaign in *Vogue*: Deborah Sherwood, Jacqui Thornton, and Nicola Davidson, "How Schoolgirl's Death Could Change the Face of Fashion," *Sunday Express*, June 2, 1996, pp. 14–15

244 Top British modeling agencies tried to recruit anorexia patient: Ibid.

Index